Allergy

A Practical Guide to Coping

Jonathan Maberly MBBS, MRCP, FRACP and
Honor Anthony MBChB

The Crowood Press

First published in 1989 by
The Crowood Press
Ramsbury, Marlborough
Wiltshire SN8 2HE

© Dr D.J. Maberly and Dr H.M. Anthony

British Library Cataloguing in Publication Data

Maberly, J.
Allergy: A practical guide to coping
1. Man. Allergies
I. Title
616.97

ISBN 1 85223 172 6

Line diagrams by Sharon Perks

Typeset by Inforum Typesetting, Portsmouth
Printed in Great Britain by MacLehose & Partners Ltd

Contents

Foreword

Allergy is a popular modern word, but unfortunately it is often misused. It can mean different things to different people. Most doctors have a rather limited definition – an abnormal reaction caused by an immunological disturbance – whilst some people use the word for things they simply dislike – 'I think I'm allergic to morning!' But many people (perhaps half of us at some time in our lives) experience unpleasant and sometimes alarming symptoms that are not immediately recognised and which at times defy scientific explanation. They are real, but are often mistaken for psychological symptoms. This is not to deny that imaginary symptoms can look like real ones, but it is grossly unfair to blame real 'organic' illness on a patient's imagination.

I welcome this book for its bold attempt to explain a difficult and complex subject. It is a self-help manual, although there are a number of references (which should be heeded) to the importance of asking your doctor's or dietician's advice before committing yourself to long-term changes of diet or lifestyle.

The authors present us with a wide spectrum of conditions which can be produced by allergic disease. Most of us can do a great deal to help ourselves, if we have a mind to do so, and need not bother our doctors at all. The guidelines presented here should help us to identify our problems, and correct our way of life if we have gone off track, without getting into difficulties. The authors have wide practical experience of their subject, and I anticipate that this book will be of immense value to many people.

If you remain doubtful, take a quick look at the last chapter. If you recognise there something which strikes a chord in your experience, then may I suggest you read carefully through the earlier chapters. Who knows – it may really change your life!

Alan Franklin FRCP DCH
Consultant Paediatrician and Allergist
St John's Hospital, Chelmsford

Introduction

Some people regard allergy as a relatively straightforward condition, giving rise to hay fever, asthma, some skin conditions, anaphylaxis and nothing else. But over sixty years ago doctors started to show that allergy or intolerance to food caused a number of other chronic symptoms. Starting in the 1920s, Dr Albert Rowe published papers on special diets in the control of all sorts of symptoms. Dr Theron Randolph then established that sensitivities to other environmental substances, including chemicals, also contributed. Other doctors joined them and at first called this approach 'clinical ecology', changing later to 'environmental medicine' to emphasise the treatment aspect. In the 1970s Dr Richard Mackarness visited Dr Randolph in Chicago, and later wrote the first British book on the subject, *Not All in the Mind* (Pan, 1976).

The timing of the development of environmental medicine was unfortunate: the last fifty years have been an age of dramatic 'high-tech' advances in medicine, particularly the development of potent drugs, offering what may seem to be an easy way out of illness. Neither the 'low-tech' discipline of observation, nor the common-sense policy of avoidance, have anything in common with the 'high-tech' developments seen as the growing points of modern medicine, although in the past most important medical advances were made by careful observation and questioning, and trying out treatments, even if the precise mechanisms were not fully understood.

Doctors generally tend to be sceptical about this interpretation of the cause of chronic symptoms, partly because of the term 'allergy' which many insist should be restricted to reactions known to be caused by one particular type of immunological mechanism. This has led to a general neglect of the subject, and even now there is very little teaching about allergic disease for doctors or medical students. In the UK allergy was only recognised as a speciality in 1986, and only a handful of consultants are recognised as specialists. This is quite inadequate for the proper management of what are relatively common and disabling chronic conditions.

As people have become aware of the wide range of symptoms caused by allergies, and have heard of (or met) patients helped by allergy management, difficulties have arisen because of their own doctors' lack of knowledge of this field. If their symptoms are somewhat unusual and nothing abnormal is found on investigation, patients are often told that the symptoms are due to stress, or are 'all in the mind'. They may be advised to put up with them, or offered tranquillisers or anti-depressants (questionable advice, now that tranquillisers are known to be addictive). Even if the patient suspects that food or the environment contributes to his symptoms, and wants to take constructive action, his doctor may not have the experience to guide him, and he is thrown back on his own resources and has to look elsewhere for help.

This book aims to explain the basic concepts of allergy, and the underlying causes of allergic disease and intolerance, and to show what ordinary people can do to help themselves. It will deal with the prevention of allergy, the simple principles of the management of allergic diseases, and precautions to take to avoid the major allergens. Generally it is about how you can improve your own health in the absence of appropriate personal medical advice. It is written as simply as is consistent with giving an accurate account of the subject, keeping technicalities to a minimum, and is based on personal experience in the field of allergy over 15 years.

If your own GP cannot help you, there may be a doctor near with an interest in allergic conditions If not, read this book, discuss it with your GP, and then carry out any suggestions that seem to apply to you, keeping him informed of your progress. If you have many fairly severe symptoms, or are disabled by symptoms, it may be unwise to apply self-help. Write to one of the allergy societies (*see* Appendix I for the addresses) to ask for the name of the nearest allergist to whom your GP could refer you: the most severe cases are best evaluated as in-patients in a controlled environment (details from the BSAEM). You need to be referred, but no one insists that your GP is wholeheartedly behind your referral. If you fail to find the help you need, you might think of writing to your MP, to your Regional Medical Officer or to the DOH: the provision of medical services is largely under central direction, and it may help them to be made aware of gaps.

1
What is Allergy?

TERMINOLOGY

Although the term 'allergy' is now used frequently, it was only coined in 1906 by von Pirquet, a Viennese physician. He described it as an altered or abnormal reaction by one or more tissues of the body after exposure to, or contact with, a foreign substance. This is a purely clinical definition. He was referring to conditions such as eczema, asthma, hay fever and urticaria (nettlerash). Since that time the immunological basis for these allergic reactions has been defined, and as more and more information has become available about the mechanisms that cause the reactions, von Pirquet's definition has come to be seen by many as insufficient. Stressing the immunological nature of the reactions is particularly import-ant since other types of reaction have also been described, based on completely different types of mechanism. For instance, the term 'intolerance' is used where it can be demonstrated that, due to biochemical idiosyncracy (an inbuilt anomaly, usually of enzyme function), there is abnormal processing of a substance, and an abnormal reaction occurs following ingestion or inhalation of that substance. A typical example is milk intolerance, due to the absence of a specific substance, the enzyme (called lactase) that breaks down the milk sugar, lactose. Lactase is present in the mucosa of the small bowel and enables the lactose to be digested and absorbed. Absence of this enzyme will produce abdominal symptoms which mimic true milk allergy, but are not due to any immune disturbance. Another example is called pseudo-allergy, the triggering of part of the immune system by a *chemical* mecha-nism; the symptoms that result again mimic genuine allergic reactions.

References to allergic diseases date from Greek and Roman times, including quite clear descriptions of asthma in Greek literature. Interestingly there is no description of hay fever (this condition appears to have been totally unknown) but food allergy, producing nettlerash reactions (urticaria), is mentioned. Relatively few records of allergic disease exist from later periods, but at the beginning of the nineteenth century accounts again started to appear. The first account of hay fever was published in 1802, the second in 1819 and the third in 1828: from then on hay fever was recognised more and more commonly, until it has now become an epidemic affecting up to 8–10 per cent of the population.

This increase is also reflected in asthma and eczema. Recent studies have shown a progressive increase in asthma, such that approximately 12 per cent of children in New Zealand now have asthma at some time before they reach the age of ten, and in the UK the incidence is similar. Eczema has shown a progressive increase over the last thirty years and now affects something like 6 per cent of the population. The increase also applies to other allergic diseases: twenty years ago allergic diseases overall were thought to affect about 6–7 per cent of the population but recent reports from the USA range from 25 to 50 per cent. Most of the symptoms are mild, but a significant number of patients suffer from symptoms that cause chronic ill health. Every year some adults and children die of allergic reactions; asthma is now responsible for between 1,500 and 2,000 deaths per year in the UK alone. So far no one has established why allergic diseases have become so common or why they still appear to be increasing in incidence, although many theories have been put forward to try and explain the phenomenon.

VIEWS ABOUT ALLERGY

There are two schools of thought within the medical profession concerning the use of the word 'allergy'. One school holds that all reactions should be proved to have an immunological basis before they can be actually classified as 'allergic'; the other that reactions that are abnormal and have the clinical characteristics of allergy should be provisionally regarded as allergic until proved otherwise. Both groups regard the standard allergies as allergic, and at the other end of the spectrum neither would regard the biochemical intolerances as such. In between these extremes are conditions which appear clinically to be allergic but are not yet accepted by the establishment (we shall use the word 'allergy' for these), and others for which there is no evidence as to mechanism.

The situation at the moment is unsatisfactory. While the controversy rages many doctors assume that if the basic tests for atopic allergy are negative, then the patient cannot possibly be suffering from an allergic reaction. As a result many patients who are suffering from genuine allergic reactions are now told that there is nothing wrong with them, and that they have to learn to live with their symptoms. They are often regarded as hypochondriacs and may be referred to a psychiatrist. As a result many of these patients go elsewhere to seek help.

MECHANISMS

It is vital for the body to defend itself from adulteration by foreign material and invasion by foreign organisms such as bacteria, parasites, fungi, and so on. The first line of defence is the structural barrier between the body and the outside world; this consists of the skin covering the outside of the body and the mucous linings separating the body from the air and particles in the respiratory tree (nose and lungs), and the contents of the gut (mouth, stomach and bowel) and of the urinary tract, all of which are exposed to foreign matter. The second line of defence is formed by the collaboration of immunological defences, scavenger cells and inflammation. These are concentrated near all the surfaces which come into contact with the external world in any form.

The immunological defences are composed of cells with special functions, and a family of antibodies, each molecule of which is formed with the capacity to recognise a foreign molecule. The foreign substances which can be recognised in this way are referred to as antigens, or allergens. Almost any compound can be an antigen – it is a functional definition. In the course of protecting the body these mechanisms may incidently cause damage to tissue, especially if antibodies of damaging type are induced in high concentration, or if substances usually excluded by the structural barrier are allowed through because of overexposure or for any other reason.

There are four main members of the family of immunoglobulins (or antibodies), and the name of each is prefixed by Ig (for immunoglobulin). IgM and IgG are the best known; when you are immunised, the aim is to produce these antibodies to protect you from infection. The role of IgA is to protect the mucous membranes from absorbing damaging foreign material, and to eliminate any food materials which are absorbed without complete breakdown before they can cause any damage. The fourth, IgE, is the type of antibody which causes atopic allergy. Some individuals (atopics) are inclined to overproduce IgE: this is useful in resisting parasites and probably in other ways but predisposes to atopic diseases, atopic asthma, hay fever, urticaria, and so on. IgE sticks to the surface of mast cells and basophils – special cells (full of potent chemical messengers) that are present in the skin, mucous membranes and the bloodstream. The messengers are rapidly released if the cell comes into contact with an allergen with the correct 'fit' for the IgE on its surface, provided that both are present in the right quantities. This is the basis of the 'immediate' reaction which is elicited by skin tests – in the skin the effects are usually complete within 10 minutes; in the blood the comparable reaction gives rise to anaphylaxis which is even quicker. It is the chemical messengers (or mediators) which effect the damage. Traditional desensitisation aims to induce the production of IgG antibodies to 'mop up' the allergen before it reaches the mast cells: it can be very effective in some people.

However, IgE reactions are only responsible for a proportion of the allergic reactions which give rise to damage or symptoms: other sorts of immunological reactions also occur and cause the release of potent chemical mediators. Reactions involving IgM or IgG antibodies may do so, causing symptoms that develop almost as quickly as those caused by IgE. Messengers may also be released when complexes (that are formed when antibodies react with antigen) are deposited in tissues, and this may be delayed for hours, even days. Other forms of reaction depend on the release of mediators when specialised cells (types of lymphocytes) recognise antigen directly; these reactions are slower still and may not reach their peak for 2–3 days; contact dermatitis is an example.

Understanding some of these facts helps you to see why the rate of onset and sites of reactions can be so variable.

The characteristics of the immune response are that antibodies 'fit', and that they are only produced *after* a significant contact with the allergen, so the first contact does not usually give rise to symptoms. These are noticed after the second, or a later, exposure; indeed, you may suddenly start to react to a substance that you have been in contact with for years. The 'fit' is referred to as the 'specificity'; an antibody is specific for a single allergen, and will only cross-react with other allergens which are very similar, usually in the same family of substances.

Because it is the chemical messengers which cause the effects, immune reactions can be mimicked by substances which have the same effect as the messengers: this is used each time a prick test is performed; a positive control with a messenger (histamine) is included to check that the skin is able to give a positive result. Mediators may also occasionally be released by other substances in what is termed pseudo-allergy.

The problem of preventing the entry of harmful substances is obviously most difficult in those organs of the body designed for absorption – for instance, the lungs (for the absorption of oxygen), and the gut (of food and water). It is no surprise that asthma, in response to inhaled allergens, should be one of the major allergic diseases. The fact that food can also be a major allergen source is equally unsurprising, but much less well recognised; it can produce asthma as well as a wide range of other symptoms. The details of the mechanisms that protect the body from damage from absorbed, incompletely-digested food are gradually being worked out: the main point to make here is that anything which disturbs the barrier efficiency of the gut tends to lead to food allergy. There are two main examples of this: gastroenteritis (particularly viral gastroenteritis) often leads to food allergy in children, and patients with food allergy tend to develop further food allergies unless they are managed effectively.

TESTING FOR ALLERGY

Because of the long-standing lack of interest in allergic reactions, relatively little work has been done on developing good accurate tests. However, one aspect has been well documented – that relating to atopy, or IgE-mediated allergy. For a long time it has been known that if you place a drop (or small piece) of a substance that the patient is allergic to on the skin and then prick through it with a needle or small blade to introduce a minute amount into the skin itself (called a *prick test*), within 10 minutes a raised wheal will appear, surrounded by a red inflammatory area. This is a typical immediate reaction produced by an interaction between IgE and the antigen. This test is used to diagnose the presence of allergy in patients who are known to have allergic symptoms. It can be used with a wide range of allergens, including house dust, house dust mite, pollens, moulds, animal dander, and many other substances, but not with any substance that might itself release the mediators. It is a useful technique, but has its limitations, since all it tells you is that there is IgE against the specific antigen in the skin of that patient; it does not tell you whether at that moment in time it is clinically significant. These tests can be backed up by blood tests measuring the total level of IgE in the bloodstream, or the level of IgE antibody against specific antigens, such as dog and cat dander. If the level of IgE is high, and specific IgE is present, it provides much stronger evidence that the patient is sensitive to those substances, but again it must be correlated with clinical history before one can be confident that that specific allergen is actually contributing to the patient's symptoms.

The prick test causes problems because many doctors rely on it to exclude the diagnosis of allergy and if the test is negative they will confidently tell the patient that they have no allergic disease. This may be untrue; prick tests in the skin are not always positive when there are IgE reactions in other tissues, and other types of allergy do not give positive prick tests. Until we develop more sophisticated blood tests to pick up the other sorts of allergic reactions, these misconceptions will continue.

A more direct but much more time-consuming approach is actually to challenge the patient with the substance concerned and note any reaction. This has the advantage of detecting reactions whatever mechanism is involved, provided that the observation period is long enough. A good example is a person who suffers from hay fever. Specific grass pollen is collected, the patient is told to sniff a small amount of the grass pollen and the reaction over the next hour or two is noted; the amount of blockage in the nose can also be measured. If a patient sniffs a grass pollen to which he is sensitive and it produces typical hay fever symptoms, he is allergic to it, provided that the conditions of the test were strictly controlled. Similarly, in asthmatics, a *bronchial challenge test* can be carried out. The patient inhales small amounts of the substance which upsets him, and the effect is followed, both on symptoms and on his ability to blow, using a peak flow meter. If the substance produces an acute asthmatic attack, this is strong evidence that it is one of the substances producing asthma in that person. These tests are laborious and time-consuming, best carried out in a laboratory, and only give answers about sensitivity to the allergens tested, with no indication about how many other allergens may be contributing to the symptoms. On occasion these tests can be dangerous, as a severe acute reaction can be produced, and at the present time only a few hospitals throughout the country are actually using them.

Oral challenge tests are frequently used to establish the presence of a reaction to certain foods. These tests are much safer to do and do not require laboratory conditions, so they can be used much more widely, except in children with eczema and babies (*see* Chapter 8). Tests performed by injecting small amounts of different concentrations of preparations of different foods into the skin are frequently used in conjunction with oral challenge testing. Some people use them as a battery without oral challenge; under these circumstances, they can suggest sensitivity, but give no indication of whether it is clinically relevant. Other people claim that tests such as the cytotoxic food test and the vega test are able to detect sensitivity, but in our view they have not been shown to give results that are reliable enough for general clinical use.

Many substances come into contact with a person's skin and certain people develop either atopic eczema, or contact dermatitis. These are two different conditions. Atopic eczema is a skin reaction that occurs in patients who are allergic to substances that they either eat, or inhale, or touch, whereas contact dermatitis specifically relates to substances the patient touches, which cause a skin reaction at that site. Over the past forty years many thousands of chemicals have been introduced into the environment which had never been present before: over 60,000 are now in everyday use (*see* Chapter 3). Certain people start to react to these chemicals, producing various types of allergic reactions, including contact dermatitis.

A very simple way to test substances when the major problem is eczema or contact dermatitis is by doing a *patch test*. This is normally carried out at the local hospital in the skin department, but simple patch testing can be carried out at home to give a rough guide as to whether you are sensitive to a certain substance or not. The technique is relatively simple. You take a small waterproof plaster with a central piece of lint, and place a sample of the substance you want to test on the lint. The plaster is then placed on the forearm, on the front surface, and left in position for 48 hours if the patch is comfortable. Following removal of the patch the area of skin is observed immediately, after one hour, and then over the next 72 hours. If a rash or a raised wheal appears, then this strongly suggests that you are sensitive to that substance. The substances used can be anything you normally come into contact with; make-up, detergents, soaps, shampoos, deodorants, hair-sprays, body lotions, and so on. Substances round the house which you might not normally think of, such as house plants, dust, materials that you wear, and medications prescribed by the doctor to treat your skin condition, can also be tested.

Any substance can be tested, but it is important to choose a concentration which simulates normal conditions. If you are testing shampoos, soaps, body lotions, and cosmetics you can use the neat substance. If you want to check your washing powder, then you should take a few drops of water from the washing machine after the soap has been added, but before the wash is carried out, or dilute the washing powder to the same extent. If you want to test plants, simply use a small piece of leaf or some of the sap. Materials are very easy: just cut a small piece of the material to be tested and fix it on the arm with the plaster. Ointments can also be tested in this way; again, these should be used neat, as they are normally put on to your skin directly from the tube.

Some of the general components in ointments or lotions may cause trouble: examples are lanolin (wool oil) and wool alcohols. These are obtained from sheep's wool and are used in a wide variety of medications, including those prescribed for skin condi-tions. As many patients who suffer from eczema or contact der-matitis are in fact sensitive to wool, the treatment tends to exacerbate their symptoms (or at the best does not produce the expected improvement). The active agent in the ointment which helps the skin condition is antagonised by the lanolin to which the patient is reacting. This can be simply tested by obtaining a small amount of lanolin from your local chemist and doing a patch test with it. Substances that contain lanolin include oilatum, frequently used as a bath emollient, E45 and other skin creams, and also a number of steroid preparations which are routinely used to treat skin problems. If you find you are sensitive to lanolin and have any doubt as to whether the substance you have been prescribed contains it, then enquire at your local chemist. He should be able to tell you whether it does or not, and also obtain an alternative preparation for you if necessary.

This is the main test that you can do youself that gives a visible result, and it is only applicable to substances that cause a reaction at the point of contact. This is not the case with many allergens. Details of how to challenge-test foods are given in Chapter 8. You can carry out simple challenge tests for other substances youself. For sensitivity to animals a good way is to stroke the animal for a few minutes and then rub one eye for 10–15 seconds: the eye will become itchy and swollen if you are sensitive. We call this the *eye test*. House dust is often tested incidently when cleaning or vacuuming the house but it can be done deliberately by sniffing some dust – the *sniff test*. This can also be applied to plants, particularly scented ones – the fact that they are scented shows that a volatile substance is being given off. Carpets and clothing with a chemical smell should also be tested in this way, in addition to using the patch test when appropriate; put a piece in a bottle, leave it sealed in a warm place for a day or two, then open it and sniff.

People who suspect that chemicals are a problem can deliberately expose themselves to the chemical under conditions that mimic normal exposure; remember that many chemicals in everyday use can be toxic. Never test any chemical at a strength at which it could burn your skin or irritate your nose or lungs. The correct exposure to use is one which would have no effect at all on normal individuals.

2
Symptoms Caused by Allergic Disease

The field of allergy is rapidly expanding, and what was thought to be relatively simple is now turning out to be very complicated. This is partly due to the increasing understanding of the immunological mechanisms causing allergic reactions, and is made more difficult by the controversy as to whether the majority of the reactions are truly allergic or not.

In 1983, Alan Scott Levin and Merla Zellerbach published a book called *The Allergy Relief Programme*, in which they divided allergic reactions into two sorts, naming them Type 1 and Type 2 reactions. Although it is not possible in every case to draw an exact line between these two types of reaction, in the present state of knowledge it is a very convenient way of looking at allergic disease, and we shall describe the types of allergy and presenting symptoms in this way. However, the terminology is unfortunate because 'Type 1' and 'Type 2' mean something different to immunologists, and could add to the misunderstandings: we shall therefore refer to them as 'Type A' and 'Type B' allergic reactions.

Type A reactions are undoubtedly allergic: Type B reactions are less well defined and may include reactions more properly described as 'pseudo-allergy' or 'intolerance'. For the sake of simplicity we will use the term 'allergy' since in our experience most respond to the same type of management as Type A reactions and can therefore best be considered as allergies for the moment.

TYPE A ALLERGY

Type A allergy is the sort of allergy that is easily recognised by most people. It often presents in very young children with the onset of typical symptoms, which may gradually get worse and peak during the teens or twenties and then slowly settle as the patient gets older. The presence of this sort of allergy can be detected by

Fig 1   Symptoms of Type A Allergy (not all specific to Type A allergy).

General symptoms	–	Anaphylaxis
Gastrointestinal symptoms	–	Vomiting, abdominal pain, diarrhoea
Skin symptoms	–	Urticaria, angio-oedema, eczema
Respiratory symptoms	–	Hay fever, rhinitis, asthma
Eye symptoms	–	Conjunctivitis

the tests used to diagnose Type A allergy which estimate the total level and specific activity of the antibody, IgE, which is always present. Type A allergy reactions come on very soon after exposure to the substance concerned (the allergen) – sometimes as quickly as 30–60 seconds after – and reach their peak within minutes; recognising the cause of the symptoms is relatively easy.

Type A allergies are typically caused by inhalants such as moulds, pollens, animal danders, and so on; less commonly they are caused by foods and comparatively rarely by environmental chemicals. Type A allergy usually involves the upper respiratory tract or nasal passages (producing hay fever and perennial rhinitis, which mimics hay fever but occurs all the year round); the lungs (producing asthma); the skin (producing eczema, urticaria (heat lumps), and angio-oedema, although only a minority of the latter are caused by Type A allergy); and in the gut (producing acute abdominal symptoms usually consisting of colic, vomiting and diarrhoea) (*see* Fig 1). Type A reactions also occur in the eye, causing conjunctivitis. This is well recognised in hay fever, but less so in relation to chronic eye symptoms from spring to autumn. Occasionally an acute generalised Type A reaction can occur, usually affecting the whole body – anaphylaxis; this is often fatal if not treated immediately.

TYPE B ALLERGY

Type B allergy is quite different. It does occur in childhood but can suddenly come on at any age. It is quite common in the teens and early twenties, rather less frequent in the later twenties and the thirties, but increases in frequency as the patient gets older. It is far more controversial because the laboratory tests are often negative, and proof that it is a truly allergic reaction is still incomplete. The causal role of environmental factors in these conditions is often unrecognised: where their role is accepted the symptoms are usually attributed to intolerance, whether to foods, chemicals or inhalants. However, in most instances there is no evidence of biochemical abnormalities giving rise to true intolerance, and we are of the opinion that most of these reactions will, in the longer term, be found to be genuinely allergic.

The typical patient who suffers from Type B allergy presents with vague symptoms that can easily be misinterpreted as being psychological in origin. Typical symptoms include lethargy, fatigue, sleepiness, night sweats, palpitations, weight fluctuation from morning to evening, and rapid weight gain or weight loss for no obvious reason. These are often associated with mild mood changes such as tension, anxiety or depression. The onset of symptoms is slow, and the duration of the reaction is quite long, so that these symptoms are rarely linked to the substances that caused them. 'Masking' can occur in a person who is reacting virtually continuously; this happens when the duration of each reaction is longer than the interval between exposures. If you are consuming a cup of coffee six times a day, and the duration of the reaction from one cup of coffee lasts eight hours, then you will have symptoms throughout the twenty-four hours; and if you gradually became sensitive, the symptoms would get worse over a period of time. Because of the long duration of each reaction there is no obvious connection with the precipitating substance. There may be low-grade symptoms most of the time which temporarily get better just after the offending food is eaten, and then get worse again. This often leads to *increased* consumption of the offending food in an attempt to get relief.

There are several other characteristics of this kind of allergy which add to the confusion. Firstly, the person does not necessarily have symptoms all the time – they may cycle. For instance, a patient may have symptoms for four, five, or six days running and then have a clear period without any symptoms: the reason for this is not understood. Secondly, the severity can fluctuate quite markedly, only partly depending on the frequency and extent of the contact with the allergen. Thirdly, if the person ceases to be exposed, he may become tolerant to the allergen after a period of time, so that re-exposure produces no symptoms. However, with exposure on a regular basis symptoms are likely to return before long and build up to their previous severity. This makes research into this sort of allergy difficult and confusing to do, since people who have been thought to be allergic to a food and have stopped eating it for a month or two may give negative test results.

SYMPTOMS OF TYPE A ALLERGY

The systems normally affected by Type A allergy are the gastro-intestinal system, the skin and the respiratory system. These are the main organs at direct risk from the environment. In the respiratory system, a very common presenting symptom is hay fever. Hay fever symptoms are not just limited to the upper respiratory tract. Most patients also develop allergic conjunctivitis at the same time, with symptoms of itching, and running and swelling of the eyes, to the extent that at times they may have difficulty in seeing. Conjunctivitis can also occur due to exposure to other substances, such as house dust mite and animals; indeed some of the most severe episodes of conjunctivitis occur after exposure to animals, which can give rise to extreme sensitivity.

Asthma is another common symptom which occurs in Type A allergy sufferers, particularly among the younger patients; in older asthma patients Type A allergy becomes much less common, and over 50 years of age uncomplicated Type A allergy is comparatively rare.

Gastro-intestinal symptoms occur quite frequently as a result of Type A allergy. The symptoms normally consist of vomiting, or abdominal pain and diarrhoea, starting rapidly after exposure to the substance concerned. This substance is usually a food, although the same sort of reactions also occur in people who are sensitive to medications – such as antibiotics and cough medicines – or to substances contained in foods or drugs, such as colourings, flavourings, and so on.

The skin can be affected in two ways. Eczema is the first condition; it is extremely common and is increasing in incidence. Eczema is not a pure Type A allergic reaction, but is more complicated. However, in many patients who suffer from eczema, especially children, Type A allergy is the dominant element. The child normally presents with itching, which at times can be intractable, and is usually much worse at night: the skin becomes thickened and then breaks down and bleeding occurs, with resulting exudation of fluid and crusting. In patients who suffer from allergy to foods, the flexures tend to be predominantly involved – mainly the front of the elbows and behind the knees. In patients who are sensitive to other substances the extensor surfaces are predominantly involved. If the eczema is severe it can spread to involve the whole body surface, although it tends to pick out specific areas which vary from person to person. Certain parts, such as the face or hands, are often spared. (The face and hands are often involved in what is called contact dermatitis, which comes on as a result of local contact with specific substances, and represents a different form of allergy – contact allergy.)

The second dominant skin symptom is diffuse swelling associated with itching, and sometimes blanching of the skin, called urticaria. The two major types of urticaria seen are angio-oedema (swelling of the deeper parts of the skin), and the less severe typical urticaria (swelling of the superficial part of the skin). Angio-oedema often involves the face, lips, tongue and throat, but can involve any other part of the body. The swelling may be so grotesque that it makes the person look quite ugly, and can be very embarrassing. It comes on acutely, and usually settles with appropriate treatment within 6–8 hours. Angio-oedema occurs quite frequently in children and less commonly in adults in response to foods, starting very quickly, even within seconds of the food being placed in the mouth. The food responsible is easily recognised and avoided. In young children it is a sign that is not always recognised; the child gets a minor swelling of the lips or tongue, which may be missed, or thought to be due to something else, and the mother goes on giving the child that food. One of two things will happen: either the child becomes tolerant and ceases to have symptoms, or the symptoms become worse until the situation becomes obvious and the child is taken off the food.

There are other kinds of angio-oedema not related to Type A allergy, often of longer duration and more difficult to treat. Some are due to enzyme anomalies, and are really pseudo-allergies.

The urticaria that occurs in Type A allergy is often quite widespread, but is limited to the superficial part of the skin. It is often extremely irritating. It tends to come on acutely and to be relatively short-lived; if the cause can be identified and eliminated, it will settle completely.

Finally, there is a comparatively rare but much more dangerous form of allergic reaction in Type A patients – anaphylaxis. This is IgE-mediated and a generalised reaction to an allergen. The commonest foods to cause this sort of reaction are the various forms of nuts, peanuts, and fish, although any food can do it. Bee and wasp stings classically cause severe anaphylactic reactions. Some medications are well known for doing it – penicillin is the one most commonly involved, but nearly all the antibiotics, and many other drugs, can sometimes cause anaphylactic reactions.

The reactions start within minutes of exposure: the symptoms are usually generalised, consisting of itching, diffuse swelling, palpitations and shortness of breath. The onset is rapid and, if the reaction is severe, the patient may become acutely ill, collapse and lose consciousness. If untreated he may die within a matter of minutes. Luckily, however, these severe reactions are uncommon and only a small number of deaths occur every year as a result of them. Less severe reactions are much more common. They are not life-threatening, but can be very frightening for the person concerned. Luckily they respond very well to medical treatment.

Similar acute life-threatening reactions can also occur without an IgE mechanism being involved: they are then known as 'anaphylactoid'. They are often caused by drugs (such as aspirin) and other chemicals. They respond to the same medical treatment.

SYMPTOMS OF TYPE B ALLERGY

Type B reactions are very common and can affect virtually any system in the body, producing a wide variety of symptoms. Many patients complain of vague symptoms. Lethargy is one of the predominant ones, but palpitations, fluid retention, sweating, poor sleep or insomnia, mood changes, weight changes, and so on, are all very commonly described by these patients. Most patients complain of a combination of symptoms, and are frequently embarrassed to admit to the large number of symptoms from which they suffer. The commonest symptoms of Type B allergy are shown in Fig 2. The wide variety of symptoms that can occur is one of the reasons why people are sceptical about this sort of allergy, and when you read the list you will understand why.

Fig 2   Some of the symptoms of Type B reactions.

General symptoms	Lethargy, inappropriate sweating, fluid retention, weight changes, obesity, difficulty in losing weight, food cravings, sleeplessness, disturbance of sleep rhythms, waking tired, mood changes, palpitations, bruising, cold hands and feet.
Respiratory and cardiovascular symptoms	Chest pain, shortness of breath, wheezing, cough, phlegm, hay fever, runny nose, nasal obstruction or crusting, catarrh, ankle swelling, swelling of the fingers or round the eyes, easy bruising, chilblains.
Mouth symptoms	Sore lips, sore tongue, oral thrush, blood blisters in the mouth, tooth abscesses, gum boils, bleeding gums, mouth ulcers, salivary gland swellings.
Gastrointestinal tract symptoms	Thirst, heartburn, wind, abdominal pain, abdominal bloating, diarrhoea or constipation [or both], itchy bottom.
Genito-urinary symptoms	(Mainly in women.) Urinary frequency, cystitis, stress incontinence, vaginal discharge including vaginal thrush, PMT, painful periods, irregularity of periods.
Nervous system symptoms	Headaches (including migraine), photophobia (light hurting the eyes), variation in eyesight or in ability to focus, sore eyes, buzzing in the ears, numbness or tingling, lack of concentration, poor memory, difficulty with speech, writing or spelling, hyperactivity (inability to relax), depression, irritability, unreasonable behaviour, aggression.
Skin symptoms	Recurrent urticaria (heatlumps), eczema, patches of flaky, dry skin, brittle nails, flaking nails, hair falling out.
Skeletal symptoms	Back ache, painful and/or swollen joints, aching and/or tender muscles, tender bones, restless legs, cramps.

Note   In children all the above symptoms may occur, but they most commonly present with severe and sudden changes of mood, aggression, growing pains, night cramps, ear infections and glue ear, hyperactivity, recurrent tonsillitis, severe nappy rash, bed-wetting, or a combination of these.

Fig 3   Illnesses which may respond to allergy management.

Hypertension, cardiac arhythmias, Reynaud's disease, arterial spasm

Oesophagitis, Crohn's disease, ulcerative colitis, irritable bowel syndrome
(irritable colon, spastic colon)

Recurrent cystitis, premenstrual syndrome

Migraine, post-viral fatigue syndrome (ME)

Some psychiatric illnesses and some cases with rheumatoid arthritis, other
types of arthritis, myalgia and 'fibrositis', including those with
considerable disability

Many of these symptoms may also be caused by other illnesses, including illnesses for which standard medical treatment is needed and is effective. When caused by allergy the symptoms are frequently multiple; they are usually chronic and often intractable and may or may not be negative to conventional investigations. They characteristically vary in severity from time to time. At present they often lead to an unjustified diagnosis of hypochondria, or even of mental illness. To most people this list of symptoms would seem so extensive as to be unlikely to result from a common cause. However, we have both seen examples of all these symptoms occurring in patients and clearing with environmental medical treatment, with the patients becoming well.

There are a number of illnesses, which are usually given other diagnoses, which may also clear with this sort of treatment (Fig 3). In some (for example, irritable bowel syndrome, and migraine when it is associated with other symptoms), good results can be expected in nearly all cases, but in others (such as rheumatoid arthritis, and post-viral fatigue syndrome (ME)) the response is less predictable. Other illnesses may have mixed causes: for instance, in certain patients cystitis may sometimes be an infection and at other times an inflammation without infection. The recommendations about personal hygiene should therefore be followed in addition to using an environmental approach. The illnesses which may respond are all chronic, may be disabling and may otherwise require long-term medication. An attempt at control using environmental medicine is worth while for any patient with these syndromes, since many of the patients who fail to show dramatic improvement get some relief and need fewer drugs.

3
Allergens and Other Triggers

There are many different substances which can cause reaction in certain individuals; the simplest way to consider them is under three headings – inhalants, foods and chemicals (Fig. 4). Many of these substances are undoubted allergens, but in this chapter the use of the term 'allergen' does not necessarily imply that an allergic role has been proved.

INHALANTS

Inhalants are substances which are dispersed into the atmosphere as fine particles, and deposited on the conjunctiva, or in the nose, throat or lungs, or on the skin. The most potent allergens tend to be proteins, although carbohydrates and fatty substances can also cause problems. Some of the particles get into the atmosphere in tiny droplets and, once dry, are dispersed by air currents: others are released as part of the reproductive cycle of plants, or moulds.

Patients with Type A allergy are most often affected by inhaled organic particles giving rise to an IgE-mediated type of reaction. Type B allergy is less frequently associated with inhalants, although it is still quite common.

Moulds

The largest group of inhaled allergens are the moulds: moulds grow on food, damp paintwork, wood, and any other organic matter such as leaves and bark, and in the earth itself. There are approximately 30,000 different moulds. When moulds reproduce they produce very fine particles called spores, which are released in very large numbers, often millions at a time, from what appears to be a relatively small amount of mould. The number of allergenic moulds is probably relatively small – so far only 30–40 moulds

Fig 4   Substances that can cause allergy, pseudo-allergy or intolerance.

Substance	Route of entry	Kinds
Organic		
Inhalants	Nose, eyes, lungs, skin	Moulds, pollens, plant sap, scent, dander, oils, mites
Foods	Mouth, gut, inhalation, bladder*, vagina and vulva*	All
Chemical		
Food additives	Mouth, gut	Colourings, flavourings, flavour enhancers, etc.
Food contaminants	Mouth, gut	Pesticides, herbicides, coating agents (waxes, oils, sprays), bulkers, drugs used to treat stock
Water contaminants	Mouth, gut, eyes, skin	Many contaminants (including chlorine); responsible agent often unknown
	Lungs	Chlorine
Drugs	Skin, eyes, mouth, gut, bladder*	Many kinds, including antibiotics
	Vagina and vulva	Topical and ingested *
Other chemicals	Skin, nose, lungs, eyes, mouth, gut, bladder*	Many kinds and sources

* during excretion, often as a metabolic product.

have been shown to be specifically allergenic as far as human beings are concerned – but it is likely that more will be recognised in due course as new techniques are developed to identify which moulds are responsible for people's symptoms.

Moulds can be seasonal, or perennial, which basically means that the spores are released into the atmosphere either during certain months of the year, or all the year round. Certain moulds are produced only in the summer, and are released between May and November. The autumn moulds are mainly the fungi such as mushrooms and toadstools, which are called *Basidiospores*. Other moulds (such as *Aspergillus* and *Penicillium*) produce spores all the year round and, although the numbers of spores released tends to vary from time to time, they can be responsible for symptoms throughout the twelve months of the year.

Sometimes spores can be present in very high concentrations: for instance, spore counts as high as 12 million per cubic metre (m^3) have been recorded when a farmer is feeding his cattle with mouldy hay; it is not surprising that a farmer who is sensitive to those spores develops symptoms under these conditions.

Fig 5   Sources of inhalant allergens.

Allergen	Where found	Kinds	Worst time
Moulds	Damp vegetation, etc.	Many	Aug/Sept
	Damp in houses Humidifiers (air conditioners) Hay and straw, mushroom farming	Many	
Pollens (light)	Anywhere while high pollen count esp. hay fields		
Grass		Many	May/July
Tree		Birch, beech, hazel, elm, ash, oak, alder, pine	Feb/June
Plants		Nettles, plantain, mugwort, etc.	Summer
Pollens (heavy)	Close to source	Chestnut, lime, etc.	Windy weather
Sap and scent	Close to source	Various	Grass and weed-cutting, hedge-trimming, oil-seed rape in flower
Organic dusts	Wood-working, baking, etc.	Wood, flour, cotton, etc.	

Animals and birds			
Dander, oil and hair	Furry animals	Various	
Faeces	Birds, small animals		
Saliva	Cat fur		Dried to powder
Urine	Especially small mammals		
Insects, etc.			
House dust mite faecal pellets	Near man, bedding, carpets, etc.	Various	Humidity and warmth, vacuuming
Storage mite	Grains		Bulk storage
Animal mites	Coats of furry animals		Contact: brush, stroke
Bees and wasps	Flowers, fruit, etc.		Summer
Mosquitoes, midges, etc.	Near water		Summer

Pollens

The next group are the pollens. Grass pollen is by far the best known and the most common. Its season extends from May to July and produces the typical hay fever symptoms that many people recognise. Pollen counts above $50/m^3$ are often associated with symptoms, and when they exceed $300/m^3$ the symptoms become severe. Peak counts can rise as high as $3–4,000/m^3$ in localised areas, and even higher when a field of hay is being harvested. Nearly all grasses are wind-pollinated, relying on the wind to carry the pollen from plant to plant: insects are not involved.

Virtually all trees, shrubs and plants produce pollen. If the plant is wind-pollinated the pollen is very light and produced in very large quantities. In windy conditions specific pollens can be carried for hundreds of miles, before they finally settle out. Typical examples of wind-pollinated trees are elm, ash, oak, beech, silver birch, hazel, and alder. Pine trees produce large amounts of wind-carried pollen, and it has been known for pollen to be carried across the North Sea from Scandinavia to the east coast of Britain. Nettles, mug-wort and plantain are examples of plants which produce large amounts of pollen; all of these have been known to produce symptoms in people allergic to pollens.

Many other plants, shrubs and trees are insect-pollinated. In this case the pollen is heavy, is produced in much smaller amounts, and is carried by individual insects from one plant to another, ensuring fertilisation. The pollen of insect-pollinated plants and trees is rarely a nuisance, unless someone comes into close proximity to the tree, or to massed plants, under windy conditions. In some cases enough pollen may released (particularly from chestnut trees or lime trees) to travel a short distance.

Other Plant Allergens

The sap of grass and of other plants may also act as an allergen, as may the volatile substances which constitute the scent of the plant or flower. Grass sap often contributes to problems that occur particlarly when grass is mown, and weed sap may also be involved.

Patients who are sensitive to grass sap may develop an urticarial rash on contact with grass, or get rhinitis, particularly when mowing the lawn. They nearly always recognise that the smell of cut grass upsets them. This explains why grass *pollen* desensitisation is not always successful. Some people are so sensitive that the smell of the uncut plant is enough to produce symptoms.

Animals and Birds

A number of patients are remarkably sensitive to animals, and this can be due to a number of different substances produced, or carried, by the animal. It is commonly thought that the hair itself is the allergen, but it is more likely that the oil on the hair is responsible for the symptoms. In the case of cats, it is the saliva that is left on the fur after they lick themselves that tends to produce the problem. Small animals (such as gerbils and hamsters) which are kept in the house all the time can produce quite severe symptoms in certain people. This is mainly due to urinary proteins which dry on the sawdust on the bottom of the cage and are then released into the atmosphere when the cage is cleaned out. Symptoms produced by these small animals can be remarkably insidious, and are often poorly recognised.

Birds such as budgerigars, parrots, pigeons, and so on, can produce potent antigens. One source of antigen is the bloom on the feathers, especially in the case of pigeons. This is a fine powder which gets on the hands when the pigeons are handled, and is released into the atmosphere. All birds excrete body proteins in their faeces, and these are released into the atmosphere when they dry on the bottom of the cage, and the cage is cleaned out. Sometimes moulds grow in the bottom of the cage, and these can also cause problems.

House Dust

House dust is and always will be with us in varying quantities. It contains numerous antigens from a variety of sources including foods, pollens, moulds, animal danders, and so on, but the most potent antigenic substances in dust are the products of house dust mites. Various forms of house dust mite have now been identified, but the two that most commonly cause problems are called *Dermatophagoides pteronyssinus* and *Dermatophagoides farinae* – splendid long names for very small creatures. They are approximately 1/5 of a millimetre long, and they thrive in the warm, humid conditions which are often present in bedding, sofas, carpets and soft toys in our very damp climate. They are found in every household in the UK in varying quantities. In a house that is damp and has the right sort of ambient temperature, dust mite concentrations can be as high as 3,000 mites per gram of dust. When the atmosphere is dry the mites cannot breed and they are present in much lower numbers. However, it is not the mites themselves that are most antigenic, it is the small faecal pellets that they produce in large numbers – up to 150 per mite each month. These faecal particles are so light that they get into the atmosphere very easily and can be inhaled or come into contact with the skin. Mites breed readily in association with feathers, wool, flock, kapok or horsehair but less with made-made fibre, foam rubber and other inorganic materials. They are found throughout the house, particularly in bedding, upholstery and carpets.

Other sorts of mites are also quite common. Grain or storage mites can cause many problems when grains are stored and transferred in large quantities from container to container. Other mites occur in straw and hay, and mites are even found in the coats of horses and other animals. In some cases of apparent animal allergy, mites (not animal products) may be the main allergen.

A number of other substances derived from living matter can be present in the atmosphere as a fine dust and cause allergic reactions; for example, cotton and wood, and other plant materials. Several give rise to well-recognised syndromes for which industrial compensation can now be paid. These syndromes include bakers' asthma from flour sensitivity, and similar conditions arising from reactions to cotton, wood dust, and so on.

FOODS

The second major group of allergens are foods. With foods Type A allergy is relatively uncommon, but when it does occur it is easily recognised, and can be extremely severe, producing anaphylaxis. It is surprising just how small an amount can cause a life-threatening reaction. In the case of peanuts, for example, the amount of peanut which could be placed on top of a pin head could cause someone to die of an anaphylactic reaction. Often very small quantities present in other foodstuffs, and hidden by processing, can produce serious and even life-threatening reactions. The commonest foods to produce anaphylaxis are the various forms of nuts, peanuts (which are in fact related to peas and beans), and seeds such as sesame seeds. Some other foods with a high protein content, such as milk, eggs or fish, have also been implicated. Sometimes people can be so sensitive that they only have to pass a shop or restaurant where the food is being cooked and inhale fumes to have a severe reaction.

Type B reactions with foods are extremely common, and can occur with any food. It has been found by experience that it is the foods consumed most frequently that are the foods most likely to cause Type B reactions. Most commonly these are the grains (mainly wheat and corn), and dairy products, sugar, tea, coffee, chocolate, potatoes, and then other foods in decreasing frequency. In our experience most food allergic people react to the foodstuff itself, but food additives can cause reactions in some. These will be considered in a later section.

Yeasts

Yeasts are very common and extremely widespread. They are present on the surface of most fruits and are responsible for natural fermentation (when foods go bad); they play essential roles in the production of alcoholic drinks, and of bread. Many foods contain yeasts in varying amounts (*see* Chapter 8); they are a good source of the B vitamins.

Allergy to bakers' and brewers' yeast is quite common. There are many other natural yeasts which do not appear to cause problems. The exception to this is *Candida albicans* which causes thrush, a condition particularly common in the young and the old, and in patients treated with antibiotics or steroids or taking the contraceptive pill. Thrush mainly affects the mouth and vagina, but occasionally there is gross infection of the gastro-intestinal tract. In most instances these conditions are all easily treated. Many doctors working in the field of clinical ecology believe that chronic low-grade infections of the bowel with *Candida albicans* can cause symptoms similar to those of allergy or intolerance. The management they use involves dietary control, nutritional supplements and anti-*Candida* drug therapy. If the patient gets better it is impossible to be certain which aspect of treatment was effective. In our experience almost all recover with good allergy management and nutritional therapy.

CHEMICALS

The third group of substances to consider are chemicals. Chemicals comparatively rarely produce Type A allergy, but commonly produce Type B reactions. Some chemicals can produce immunological reactions in their own right; others can only do so when firmly fixed to a protein or other complex molecule. At present there is little evidence that Type B reactions caused by chemicals have an immunological mechanism, and many people therefore refer to them as intolerance. However, the range of Type B symptoms caused by chemicals almost completely overlaps that caused by foods, and similar methods of management are effective whether the symptoms are caused by inhalants, foods or chemicals. It is therefore reasonable to suppose that some at least may act through similar mechanisms.

Very few people are aware of how many chemicals now pollute our environment, whether in the home, at work, at school, or outside. Chemicals are now frequently found contaminating the food we eat, the water we drink, and the air we breathe (Fig 6). It is only comparatively recently that chemicals have been produced in large amounts and released into the environment. The first chemicals produced in quantity appeared during the Industrial Revolution with the use of coal, and rapid expansion in the production of chemicals really only dates from 1945. Throughout the period from 1965 to 1978, new compounds were reported in the scientific literature at the rate of approximately six thousand a week, and this is continuing. There are now about four million different chemicals in the American Chemical Society's register and something like sixty to seventy thousand chemicals are in everyday use. The use of chemicals has infiltrated every aspect of our life and our environment. We have literally cocooned ourselves in chemicals, and over four hundred toxic chemicals have been identified in human tissues. Chemicals can all produce toxic reactions if they are present in sufficient concentration, but regulations keep most chemicals under partial control, and gross toxic reactions are relatively uncommon. Chronic non-specific long-term effects are difficult to detect.

Most people spend much of their lives being exposed to many different chemicals without being aware that they can cause any problems. When someone becomes intolerant or allergic to a chemical, they react to a much lower concentration; for instance, to the ambient concentration of a chemical which leaves other people unaffected. Reactions to chemicals produce a multitude of symptoms, similar to those from food allergens but with a greater tendency to give symptoms that could be classified as psychological, rather than physical, as the brain is predominantly affected. Symptoms such as lack of concentration, fatigue,

Fig 6   Some chemicals which cause reactions.

Chemical	Where found
Formaldehyde	*Outgasses from*: plastics, urea formaldehyde foam and glue, compressed boards, carpets *Also in*: preservatives, deodorants, personal toiletries, throat lozenges *Also used in*: bulk meat transport, moth proofing, crease resistance, sugar processing, printing
Phenol (Carbolic acid)	Soft plastics, ink, medications, perfumes, photographic solutions, herbicides, pesticides, detergents, dyes, wallpaper paste
Ethanol	Methylated spirit, surgical spirit, liqueurs, perfumes, medications, hand lotions, solvents (aerosols, etc.), paints and varnish, photographic film
Turpentine	Polishes, paints, pine furniture, flooring, etc. Christmas trees
White spirit	Paints and paint thinners, varnish
Glycerine	For sweetening and preserving food, manufacture of cosmetics, perfumes, inks, certain glues and cements, soaps, creams, suppositories
Gas, methane	(Natural gas) Gas cookers, gas boilers, gas fires and heaters
butane	Calor gas, portable gas heaters
Nitrates	Tap water
Nitrites	Preserved meats, bacon, etc., tap water
Sulphur dioxide	Atmosphere, power stations, wine-making, dried fruit, sprayed on salads to keep fresh, preservative on shrimps and shellfish
Ammonia	Cleaning agents, bleaches
Chlorine	Tap water, bleaches, swimming baths
Mixtures	
Tobacco smoke	Smoking (higher with recirculated air)
Diesel exhaust	Near heavy traffic, in cars, buses, trains, boats, etc., oil-heating
Petrol exhaust	In cars, near heavy traffic, in buildings with garage under or attached
Newspaper print	Newspapers, magazines and books

behaviour changes, irritability, tension, panic attacks, and unexplained depression, occur in patients who are allergic to foods but are more common in those who are reacting to chemicals, although other symptoms occur as well.

Types of Chemical

What chemicals do we normally come into contact with, without necessarily realising it? In the home, formaldehyde, which is present in many furnishings and fittings, and is used as a moth-proofing agent, is frequently a problem; as are fumes from the gas stove, and chemicals released with the use of aerosols, cleaning agents, detergents, polishes, perfumes, bleaches, and so on. Plastics are now widely used in the home; soft plastics are produced from phenolic substances, and phenol can be a major problem. Cigarette smoke is present in many homes, offices, theatres, and can be harmful to both smokers and non-smokers.

Outside, car and diesel exhaust fumes are present wherever there is traffic. Sulphur dioxide is another chemical which is widely distributed; it is mainly produced from power stations, but also actually used in the production of wine (especially by amateur winemakers) and dried fruit, and in the soft drink industry. It is one of the causes of acid rain, and is now universally present in the northern hemisphere. Another common problem is newspaper print. Most people read newspapers virtually every day, as well as magazines and books, and the chemical smell given off by newspapers, once recognised, is surprisingly commonly encountered.

Other major sources of chemical pollution are the fumes given off by decorating materials – paint, varnishes, emulsions, glues, and so on. Many people develop minor headaches or nausea when they come into contact with fresh paint, or varnish, but they just assume that this is perfectly normal and take no notice.

Air-fresheners are now used more and more, as if natural smells from the home have become taboo. We now see air-fresheners in the form of aerosols and solid tablets in cars, houses, offices, and public places. They are even inserted into so-called 'air filters' that can be used in the home, and some modern vacuum cleaners have them on the outlet, so that the air coming out of the vacuum cleaner smells 'nice'. The 'air-freshener syndrome' was described in an article published recently – people became quite confused and disorientated when they were exposed to the chemicals which are released from any form of air-freshener.

Indoor pollution is made worse by the modern techniques of insulating houses with double or triple glazing, total draughtproofing, and by the absence of any form of fireplace. This results in a steady increase in the concentration of chemicals within the building as a direct result of the decrease in ventilation. This is particularly serious where modern heating or ventilation systems are employed, many of which re-circulate 90 per cent (or more) of the air. In Canada and North America, people are becoming seriously concerned at the level of chemicals that occurs in these buildings as a result, and it is becoming recognised that physical illness may occur as a direct result of the chemical exposure.

This problem is particularly serious in modern office buildings where a large number of chemicals are released from photocopying machines, automatic copying paper, printing machines, and so on, and from the toiletries of the occupants of the office (perfumes, hair sprays, deodorants, body lotions, after shave). Tobacco smoke, and the residual cleaning agents from the laundering or dry cleaning of clothing add to the pollution. It is not surprising that papers have recently been published reporting a so-called 'sick building' syndrome, with as many as 55–60 per cent of the workers within these buildings becoming chronically ill, especially later in the day. Their performance progressively drops, with a marked reduction in the overall output of work from the building. This has not yet been pinned down to any specific substance, but we suspect it is due to multiple chemical pollution inducing intolerance and allergies.

Food Additives

Over 3,000 chemicals are added to foods during processing and production for human consumption. Some of the additives permitted in the UK are not allowed in other countries; for example, of 16 artificial colours allowed in the UK, each is banned by at least one other country, some by most European countries, Canada and the USA. The admissability of any compound is based on the absence of significant evidence of toxicity, mainly in animal studies, up to concentrations substantially higher than those at which they will be used. This may not be sufficient to ensure that there will be no longer-term toxic effects. Still less does it protect against allergic or intolerant reactions, which characteristically occur in sensitised or susceptible individuals only, and at concentrations very much lower than those causing toxic reactions.

Additives are used for cosmetic reasons (as colourings, flavourings, sweeteners, flavour enhancers, texture modifiers), as preservatives (including anti-oxidants), and as processing aids (to ensure that colours mix evenly, to prevent the food sticking to the container, to extract caffeine from coffee, and so on). Some additives are clearly acceptable; for instance, E170 is calcium carbonate and E330 is vitamin C – both occur naturally and both are needed. However, others are complex synthetic chemicals, used for purposes that cannot be considered necessary. Most additives have by law to be declared on the label of packaged food (not unwrapped food, or takeaways), but this is not the case with flavourings, and modified starches (for which the general title is sufficient), or processing aids, which need not be declared at all. Moreover, the final product does not need to detail substances added to one of the ingredients in a previous manufacturing process, so that packaged bread does not need to list flour additives. Many of the colourings (specifically the azo-dyes including tartrazine) have been linked with hyperactivity in children, monosodium glutamate with 'Chinese Restaurant syndrome', and other additives with asthma. Individual patients also have trouble with many others.

There has been a very healthy trend in the last few years towards decreasing the number of chemicals added to foods, and a growing number of foods are now advertised as colouring-free, additive-free or preservative-free. This has been almost entirely as a result of public disquiet and public demand, not government action. However, the label 'natural', which is increasingly being used, may not mean 'safe'. Natural colours may also be allergens, and some 'natural' colours are apparently synthetic copies. It is to be hoped that public pressure will continue until chemicals added to foods are reduced to the minimum consistent with bacteriological safety. (For more about additives *see* Further Reading.)

Food Contaminents

Foods, both animal and plant in origin, are increasingly contaminated by the residues of pesticides and herbicides used to increase crop yield and to attain the visual perfection of fruit and vegetables that producers think the public wants. The use of herbicides and pesticides now amounts to several hundred million gallons a year in the UK alone. In some cases foods may be sprayed as many as twenty to thirty times before they reach the customer. Some of the chemicals form a surface coat: these include sprays used to prevent infestation of bulk stores of grain (which particularly pollute the bran), the wax coating on citrus fruit (which may get into foods when the rind is used either in drinks or in cooking), and the mineral oils and sulphur dioxide used on ordinary commercial supplies of dried fruit.

Other sprays are systemic, that is, they depend for their activity on being absorbed into the tissues of the plant and remaining present for considerable periods. Recent legally-binding controls over the use of pesticides require that growers obey the instructions on pesticide containers (including those on the length of time that should pass after spraying before the crop is harvested). However, residues will be carried over to the food even if these recommendations are observed, and, as things stand, there is no way of ensuring that they are enforced.

Some patients are able to tolerate vegetables, fruit and/or grains from organic sources, but react to the same foods from standard commercial sources, indicating that reactions to the pesticides and/or herbicides or other contaminents are occurring.

There is no certainty that the continued use of the permitted chemicals is safe in the long term, even for non-allergic individuals. The case of DDT is instructive. DDT was widely used for years before it was realised that it was building up alarmingly in the food chain, and it was banned in the UK and the USA. However, it is still widely used in the developing world, and the UK and other countries export it for use there. As foods are imported from these countries without adequate checks it will be a long time before it is eliminated from our food chain: it takes a very long time to bio-degrade.

Meat and poultry may be contaminated by contaminents in the feed (such as herbicide and pesticide residues), by chemicals added to the feed (like the common addition of bacitrin to poultry meal in some areas), by veterinary treatment of the animal, and by treatments applied to the carcass. At one time penicillin and

37

tetracyclin were used as growth promoters in pigs and chickens: this was stopped some years ago, but other antibiotics are still permitted. Moreover, intensive husbandry leaves animals and birds subject to frequent infections (particularly with *salmonella*) and infestations, and antibiotics and other drugs are permitted for therapeutic use. With intensively-housed stock it is usually necessary to treat them all in order to prevent re-infection or re-infestation. Regulations lay down the minimal interval between treatment and slaughter for the table, but the regulations in the UK do not seem to be adequate to protect people who react to these drugs or their products.

Some other people who are sensitive to corn or to fish when they eat it themselves, find that they are unable to tolerate poultry fed respectively on corn or fish-meal. This is presumably because of detectable antigens carried over from the feed. Food may also be contaminated from wrappings, particularly from soft plastics, and from aluminium pans and containers.

Tap Water

The water supply provides yet another source of chemical pollution. Water supplies are increasingly contaminated from three main sources. The first is the intentional addition of aluminium salts (currently suspect in relation to early senility), chlorine and fluoride during water treatment. Because there is no compelling evidence that these chemicals are harmful, they are believed to be safe, and the possibility that they may be causing harm in their own right is ignored. Secondly, there is the pollution that arises from the recycling of water in big cities, particularly London. Trace chemical contamination from chemicals used in all sorts of processes gets into the land water. Most of it is not removed during recycling, but will gradually and relentlessly build up. In one major city in the USA 2,000 chemicals were identified in low concentration in the public water supply and other reports suggest that the real figure could be substantially higher than this. In the UK 160 different chemicals were identified in a sample of water in Essex, and there may have been many more present, undetected by the limited range of tests performed. The third source of pollution is the increased application of chemical fertilisers to agricultural land, much of which drains off into the land water. In some parts of this country nitrates in the water supply already exceed the maximum level recommended by the European Community, and the situation will get progressively worse over the next 10–15 years as the nitrates filter down through the water tables. In the late 1990s it is predicted that many of the water supplies in the UK will exceed the European Community regulation level. Water is also being increasingly polluted by the residues of pesticides and herbicides, applied in increasing quantities. They are present in relatively low concentrations but proving that these levels are safe is impossible. It is only recently that people have begun to realise that they may be drinking potentially harmful amounts of these substances.

Many of our patients have fewer symptoms if they drink spring water, and their symptoms recur if they go back to tap water. There is, therefore, some justification for including tap water under the title 'Allergens and Triggers' although there is no evidence to date as to the nature of the agents that are responsible, or of the mechanisms.

Overall it is a depressing picture when you take into account the pollution occurring in the atmosphere, in water supplies, and in food. We must hope that, as governments become aware of the problems, measures will be taken to reduce the number of chemicals released into the environment. Some people claim that chemical contamination has a wider significance; that the increased chemical load is responsible for the increase in allergies. They believe that patients with allergies recover more quickly if they keep their chemical load to a minimum by restricting the use of all chemicals, drinking spring water from a good source, and eating organic produce. There is no clear evidence for these claims at the present time, but if they are right, it is not surprising that the incidence of allergies is increasing.

4
Preventing Allergies

The incidence of allergy is rising. Estimates of the frequency vary, but have been gradually increasing over the years and currently range from as low as 10 per cent to as high as 50 per cent of the population. In spite of this we still know very little about why allergy occurs.

INHERITED TENDENCIES

There is no doubt about the genetic component. Between 15 and 25 per cent of the population are said to be atopic, but the term is difficult to define. The simplest way is to say that anyone who has one or more positive skin tests, on simple prick testing, is atopic. The second definition is a clinical one; anyone who suffers from a combination of at least two conditions out of the four – asthma, eczema, hay fever and urticaria – is atopic. Some doctors insist on a rigorous definition based on blood investigations, and define atopy as a genetic predisposition to produce too much IgE and therefore also to develop allergic disease. Combining these three definitions gives a realistic view of what atopy means. The actual incidence of the atopic trait also appears to be increasing. Some years ago it was thought to affect approximately 15 per cent of the population, but more recent estimates are as high as 25 per cent. Does this reflect a true increase in the genetic trait, or is its expression influenced by environmental factors? We do not really know.

Currently, approximately 75 per cent of the atopic subjects develop allergic disease, and a rough prediction can be made of the likelihood of a child being allergic by looking at the parents' history. If neither parent is atopic then only 15 per cent of the children will be atopic, and 10 per cent will develop allergic disease; if one parent is atopic, then 33 per cent of the children will have the atopic trait and about 25 per cent will become allergic; but if both parents are atopic then two-thirds of the children will be atopic, and 50 per cent will actually develop allergic disease. The incidence of allergic disease is also higher if other relatives are allergic as well. Why is this important? Is the development of allergic disease preventable? Well, there is evidence to suggest that it is and if we are going to make an attempt to prevent allergic disease occurring we need to know how big a risk there is of each child developing allergic disease in the first place, to judge how much action is appropriate in that case. If neither parent is atopic you can say 'Well, there is not a lot of chance of the children becoming allergic and precautions are not particularly called for.' However, if both parents are, then there is a very good reason for taking every precaution to try and prevent the children developing allergic disease in due course.

MEASURES FOR PREVENTION

There is no conclusive proof of the effectiveness of measures to reduce the risk of allergic disease, but what evidence there is (from experiments in animals, and some human experiments as well) suggests that there are two major groups of measures which are likely to help. One is concerned with the environment, the other with nutrition – the nutrition of the parents before the baby's conception and of the mother during pregnancy and lactation, and of the child during early childhood. The most important steps concerning prevention need to be taken before and soon after birth; we shall consider both aspects together, over the period from 6 months before the child is conceived, to when the child is at least one year old.

Animal breeders select the best animals to breed from and then feed them with first-class food, making sure there is no nutritional deficiency. Human beings tend to breed at random, and no notice is taken at all by the public or the medical profession of the nutritional adequacy of parents before they decide to have children. It is assumed that the modern diet in the Western world provides adequate nutrition for both parents. Recent evidence suggests that this is not true, and experiments have shown that mild deficiencies of vitamins or minerals are far more common both in children and in adults than had been previously thought.

For example, take the results of two recent studies; in one, school-children were put on a simple vitamin/mineral supplement and showed marked improvement in their IQ and school performance; in the second, in the USA, delinquency and aggression were significantly reduced when teenagers were put on to a better diet, avoiding junk foods, tea, coffee, sugar and so on. Another American study showed that approximately 15 per cent of high school children were verging on vitamin B_1 deficiency, and 25 per cent had a vitamin B_1 intake less than the recommended daily requirement as established in the USA.

Before Conception

Ideally, parents planning to have a family should start sorting out their diet 6 months before conception and, if necessary, take low-dose vitamin and mineral supplements throughout this time to make sure that there are no deficiencies present when conception occurs. In the father's case, at least 6 months is necessary, as the spermatozoa that fertilise the ovum at conception start to develop 3 months earlier. If you allow 3 months for the supplements to work, the man should start to take them 6 months before intended conception. In contrast, the egg starts to develop only about 10 days before it is shed, so 3 months' preparation should be adequate for the woman, unless she has been taking the Pill, when a longer period is preferable, using a barrier method of contraception, and vitamin/mineral supplements.

Other aspects of the parents' health must also be looked at. The development of the child may be adversely affected by smoking before the birth, either by the mother or the father. Smoking should be stopped and alcohol consumption reduced to a minimum, or preferably stopped. All drug therapy should be reviewed, as certain drugs may be toxic in pregnancy. Ideally, all drugs should be stopped about 6 months before conception, as we do not know enough about their action to be confident that there can be no deleterious effects at all. In addition, in our polluted environment it is well worth while thinking about the presence of toxic minerals, insecticides and herbicides. At the moment there are no readily applicable ways of estimating the true levels of pesticides, herbicides and other complex chemicals in the body, but hopefully techniques will soon be developed which will allow us to do so more easily and with greater accuracy. Recent studies have shown that if the mother has high levels of insecticide and/or herbicide in her body these may be transferred to the foetus, and more particularly after birth, when considerable amounts are passed to the child in the breast milk. This is no argument against breast feeding; cows are also exposed to these substances and presumably pass them on in their milk. The presence of simple chemicals such as lead, cadmium and mercury can, and should, be checked, as these tend to be passed on to the foetus during pregnancy, and can be quite toxic. If your own doctor cannot help you with preconceptual care and investigations, these can be arranged through 'Foresight' (*see* Appendix I).

Attention to all these matters may also help fertility. The health of the father and in particular smoking by the father is very important in this respect and is often overlooked.

Any woman who has a background of allergy should examine her diet well before she becomes pregnant, to make sure that she does not have any intolerance to foods in her normal diet. This could be done with a simple exclusion diet such as the Stone Age Diet described by Dr Mackarness (*see* Chapter 8). If she discovers that she is allergic or intolerant to certain foods, avoiding these may aid conception, and is important during pregnancy and lactation.

The First Three Months of Pregnancy

From conception to 3 months the foetus grows extremely fast, its weight increasing by a factor of at least two million. During this period it develops from an egg to a fully developed foetus with every organ formed. Obviously, this is an extremely critical time for the future child, but antenatal care does not usually start until about 3 months, and soon afterwards checks are made to see whether the foetus is grossly abnormal. Apart from the general warnings about smoking, and about avoidance of drugs and X-rays by women who may be pregnant, no active steps are taken routinely to give advice on nutrition, healthy habits, and so on during this vital early period. It would be far better to act before pregnancy starts and take more precautions, and so reduce the chances of the foetus being abnormal to an absolute minimum.

Experiments in rats and mice have shown that minor vitamin deficiencies at this critical stage in pregnancy result in the production of grossly abnormal young: with more severe vitamin deficiency the animals become infertile and produce no offspring (for instance *see* Pottenger, Further Reading). Obviously one needs to be careful in extrapolating animal results to human beings, but the experience gained during and after the end of World War II suggests that similar effects do occur. Women suffering from sever malnutrition generally failed to become pregnant, and conceptions occurring during moderate malnutrition showed an increased incidence of abnormal babies. If the development of the child is abnormal, the immune system is likely to be affected, and allergies more common. Moreover, deficiencies of certain minerals (such as zinc) in animals produce profound effects in the first generation offspring, sometimes continuing in subsequent generations. All this makes it clearly logical to recommend vitamin and mineral supplementation, and a good diet, to mothers during the first 3 months of pregnancy.

Later in Pregnancy

From 3 months to 9 months *in utero* the child continues to develop but during this time development consists mainly of growth and maturation. The immune system is developing and maturing and starting to produce its own antibodies. It has now been shown that certain mothers appear to transfer intact antigens to the foetus; these may result in the child being allergic at birth. Measurements of IgE in the cord blood after birth have also been shown to correlate with the incidence of allergy later on. In a few children, skin tests may be positive within a few days of birth, usually to egg or milk.

If the mother finds she is allergic or intolerant to certain foods, then it would be wise to avoid these foods totally during pregnancy, or at least to reduce their consumption markedly (certainly avoiding eating them every day) in the hope that the chance of sensitising the baby will be reduced. Obviously, if milk and dairy products are involved, a calcium supplement should be taken during pregnancy, to make up for the reduced intake in the diet. Fish and carob are also both first-class sources of calcium.

During pregnancy smoking should be avoided completely. The babies of mothers who smoke tend to be smaller than those of non-smokers, to have a higher incidence of hyperactivity and of allergy, and to have about twice as many respiratory infections in the first year of life. These babies are born 'small for dates', which suggests an increased chance of their immune system being affected, contributing to the risk of allergy developing later on.

After Birth

When the child is born it suddenly goes from a totally secure environment, which is free from all pathogens and largely free from allergens, to one that contains bacteria, viruses, and other infective organisms, and all the allergens which are present in the home. Unless it is exclusively breast-fed it is exposed at the same time to large quantities of a substance which is highly allergenic, and totally foreign – cow's milk and its derivatives, such as powdered milk. This is one of the most critical periods in the child's life when it suddenly has to adapt to a new environment; it has to start producing its own immune protection and it has to cope with many foreign substances with which it has never come into contact before. Breast-feeding during this period is vital.

If you go back to studies of the 1940s and 1950s, it was shown very clearly that breast-feeding had a marked protective influence on the child. There were far fewer infections of all sorts in the child, particularly gastro-enteritis, and there was also evidence of a marked decrease in allergic disease. Recent studies have not shown this obvious difference and it is difficult to explain why. One possible reason is that many breast-fed babies are given an artificial feed soon after birth, sometimes without the mother's knowledge, and this may have interfered with more recent studies. Secondly, modern milk powder preparations are far less allergenic than previously and are better balanced nutritionally. Thirdly, bottle-feeding has been used extensively in our society for about a hundred years. One of the results of this may be that many more women are now allergic, and, because they are allergic, they are less effective in preventing food allergens reaching the foetus, and/or the child via the breast milk.

Ideally, breast-feeding should be carried on for a minimum of

6 months without giving any supplements at all. The most pernicious supplement is that often given soon after birth 'to give the mother a rest'. This supplement may consist of cow's milk powder, or glucose which is derived from corn (maize), and may be the specific sensitising dose that causes the allergy, or predisposes to it. Weaning should not be started under 6 months if possible; if it becomes necessary, because the mother is not producing enough milk, or the child is becoming very hungry, then a heat-treated form of milk should be used, because high temperatures alter the allergenic proteins in the milk. Use either evaporated milk or the most processed form of cow's milk powder, introducing it as a supplement (with partial breast-feeding continued whenever possible). The child should be weaned on to the least allergenic foods to start with (*see* page 47), and only introduced to the more allergenic foods when at least 9 to 12 months old.

At birth the child's digestive system is relatively poorly developed, and is only really competent to deal with breast milk. The immune system is also still developing. Neither of these systems are ready to cope with other foods such as cow's milk, cow's milk powder, or corn syrup or dextrose. The baby is designed to have breast milk only for at least 3 months (probably 6 months or even longer), and was not meant to have any other food before this time. It has been shown that colostrum contains many components, including substances which cause the mucosa of the digestive system to mature more quickly, and a substance called 'closure factor' which acts to seal the surface of the bowel, preventing the absorption of certain foodstuffs. Colostrum also contains immunoglobulins to protect the gut, and other substances which aid the absorption of the essential minerals and vitamins from the breast milk. These substances are essential for the best development of the child's digestive system. Development will occur without them but the chances of allergy occurring are higher.

It is often suggested that young babies that are breast- or bottle-fed should be given supplements of vitamins or iron. This is not normally necessary if the mother's nutrition is adequate, and in the breast-feeding mother it is far better to give the mother the supplements and let her pass on the appropriate amount to the child, than to give the child the supplements. This is particularly so in the case of iron. Iron given to the child whilst it is breast-feeding encourages the growth of bacteria, and can cause a chronic infection in the small bowel with malabsorption of food increasing the possibility of food allergy. Apart from this, gastro-enteritis is rare in breast-fed babies; in one study, published in the late 1960s, bottle-fed babies had an incidence of gastro-enteritis 400 times that of the breast-fed babies. Following gastro-enteritis, it is not unusual for temporary food intolerance to occur, especially to wheat or milk. It is probable that children who have recurrent bouts of gastro-enteritis have an increased chance later of developing allergy to the solid foods they were taking at that time.

Weaning

About 6 months seems to be the best time to wean the child off the breast and on to solid foods. Certain foods are less allergenic than others, although all foods have the potential to cause food allergy. The best foods to start giving a child on weaning are vegetables and fruit. These should be started as simple fresh foods, peeled and liquidised or cooked as necessary. Once the child is established on these, the next food to be introduced is meat, followed by grains such as rice, and then wheat, corn, oats and so on, until finally, and not before the child is a year old, eggs, milk and fish can be introduced. It is unwise to introduce these foods under a year old, especially when there is a history of allergy either in the parents or in the siblings. Soya milk is often advocated throughout this time; this was originally because it was not a commonly-eaten food, and studies done in the 1950s showed a substantial reduction in the incidence of allergy in those taking soya milk rather than cow's milk. However, soya is now present in many commercially-produced foods and widely used in the diet, so that it no longer has this advantage and is really no better than cow's milk. It should only be used when there is cow's milk intolerance or allergy, and a hypoallergenic alternative has not been prescribed.

ENVIRONMENTAL FACTORS

Another factor that has to be taken into account is the child's environment during the first year of its life. Studies have shown that substances present in the child's environment may cause the child to become allergic if it is exposed to them during the early months of life. Children born early in the year, between January and March, show an increased incidence of hay fever, being exposed to the higher pollen levels in June and July, 3 to 6 months after birth. Children born in the middle of summer have an increased incidence of house dust mite allergy as they are exposed to increased levels of house dust mite during the autumn months, again in the same critical period of their development. Extrapolating from these studies it would seem logical that, if the child is in danger of becoming allergic, its environment should be kept as clean of potential allergens as possible during the first year. Contact with animals should be avoided completely, bedding should be of non-allergic materials, and other aspects of the home should be looked at very carefully – for instance, making sure that carpets on which the child will lie or crawl regularly do not smell strongly of chemicals. The use of chemicals in the home should be kept to an absolute minimum; aerosols, sprays, and so on, should not be used in the presence of the child, if used at all; no one should smoke in the vicinity of the child, and, preferably, neither parent should smoke at all. It has been shown that a child who has been brought up in the presence of an adult who smokes 20 cigarettes a day may be inhaling the equivalent of one to two a day.

Once the child is a year old it is much less clear how much the chance of becoming allergic is affected by environmental influences, although it would seem sensible to keep the child away from contact with animals for the first two to three years of life, to continue avoiding highly allergenic foods as much as possible (especially if there is a substantial risk of the child becoming allergic), and to make sure that the child eats a wide variety of foods so as to avoid repetitive eating. Additives, tea, coffee, and junk foods should be totally excluded from the child's diet, and sugar should be avoided; sugar is quite unnecessary for children, and may be harmful. At present there is no evidence that a child on a good balanced diet requires vitamin or mineral supplements; however, there is a need for studies to investigate whether such supplements are really unnecessary, or whether a child who has a history of allergy in the family would benefit from nutritional supplements for the first two or three years after weaning.

LATER LIFE

We do not know for certain what causes or precipitates allergic disease later in life, but experience suggests some precautions which people from allergic families might wisely take. The first again concerns diet. A varied diet should be eaten, making sure that no one food, or few foods, predominate. Rethinking food habits to avoid eating the same foods regularly every day makes an important contribution to achieving this. Bingeing should be avoided, and food cravings investigated as they are often the first sign of food allergy.

The second recommendation concerns the environment. Do not smoke; do not use unnecessary chemicals either in personal toilet or in the home; avoid aerosols, sprays and air fresheners (*see* Chapter 6); be meticulous about the appropriate use of protective clothing, ensuring ample ventilation when having to use chemicals, and washing thoroughly afterwards; and consider the out-gassing properties of household materials when planning alterations to the fabric or furnishings of your home. Be particularly careful about the bedroom and any other room in which you spend a lot of time (*see* Chapter 6). If you clean up your home your overall contact with chemicals will be substantially reduced and occasional mild exposure elsewhere can be ignored, unless cleaning up your environment reveals that you are intolerant to one of the chemicals, when you may need to avoid it if you are to remain symptom-free. Otherwise, the aim is just general reduction, not avoidance, and it is a great mistake to become fanatical about it.

Thirdly, take your health seriously, but not too seriously. Although stress is not a *cause* of symptoms due to allergy, it does seem to be a precipitating factor. Do not be surprised if you develop many allergic symptoms if you consistently drive yourself far too hard, all round the clock, or if you are (or have been) up against severe prolonged unavoidable stress. If you are in this position, yoga or relaxation may help to protect you, and it is particularly important for you to make a point of arranging to participate in activities you enjoy regularly (either relaxing activities or ones using a very different kind of concentration), to take regular exercise, and to avoid a repetitive diet.

5
Finding the Cause of Your Symptoms

If you are trying to cope with allergic symptoms, and to control them yourself, the most important step is to identify which allergens are responsible. This is difficult to do unless you are aware of the full range of allergens that may cause trouble (*see* Chapter 3). Having learned about them, you can set about finding out which are relevant for you. If you are a Type A reactor, then you have probably already identified the cause of your symptoms, or have a very good idea of where to look. If you are a Type B reactor, or a Type A reactor with additional symptoms, things are very different. The effects of the allergens will probably be masked and you are likely to be reacting to several different allergens simultaneously, which makes your task much more difficult. However, as a Type B reactor you have probably had symptoms for years and if you succeed in getting rid of them the reward will be considerable.

In this chapter we will try to show you how to set about finding the allergens you are reacting to, but remember that you are going to need professional help if you are very unwell, or if simple investigations give confusing results. Remember too that your symptoms may be caused by a physical illness which can (and should) be put right by standard treatment, for example, surgery. Make sure that your doctor is satisfied that your symptoms are not caused by any disease before you start your investigation. This does not mean that you should not investigate the possibility that allergy is contributing to your symptoms, if your doctor has given them a name and is offering you symptomatic treatment. Many of the conditions which are often managed by symptom relief may be relieved if the cause is identified using the approach of environmental medicine. If you are taking medication from your doctor you should discuss with him/her whether it would be all right to stop it. From an allergy point of view it is better not to be taking any medication while you sort out your allergies, since the drugs

Fig 7   Most likely causes of a few symptoms.

Car sickness	Petrol or diesel fumes
Sea sickness	Diesel fumes
Food craving	Foods
Inability to lose weight	Foods, chemicals
Lack of concentration, mood changes, panic attacks	Chemicals
Bloating, diarrhoea and constipation	Foods

themselves, or the other substances they contain (such as colourings, flavourings, bulking agents, gum, and so on) can sometimes be the offenders. However, as there are some drugs which should not be stopped, this should be clarified with your doctor before you start.

The first thing to realise as you set off on your detective hunt is that the things you react to may not be what you expect. Abdominal symptoms *usually* come from food allergens, but not always; nasal symptoms *may* be caused by foods or chemicals as well as inhalants, particularly if they occur out of the pollen season; migraine or lethargy, and in fact any of the other symptoms, *may* be caused by foods, inhalants, or chemicals. We will try to point out which you should think of first, but everyone is different and your aim will be to find out the cause of *your* symptoms. Some of the more consistent links with symptoms are shown in Fig 6.

Always remember that withdrawal symptoms (*see* Chapter 8) can occur when a substance that has been unsettling you is removed from your diet or environment. This may give rise to nausea, vomiting, diarrhoea, headache, aches and pains in muscles or joints, or other symptoms. If this occurs you are almost certainly on the right track. These symptoms usually last 3–5 days, and rarely more than 10 days. If they persist, you should consider the possibility that you have inadvertently introduced something that upsets you in the changes you have made.

The first step is to think about your symptoms: is there anything that makes them worse or better? Think fairly widely, remembering that some reactions come on very quickly, but that others may be delayed for 1 or 2 days, or sometimes longer. Paradoxically, either effect (worse or better) is likely to be significant. The person who eats chocolate to relieve persisent migraine is probably allergic to chocolate, and chocolate is a cause of the migraine. Is there any time of day, or of the week, when your symptoms are worse? Do they vary with the seasons, or with the weather? Are you better or worse when you go on holiday and, if so, does it depend on where you go? If you improve on holiday in a warm, dry climate and relapse on your return home you are almost certainly sensitive to chemicals or inhalants. If you get worse on holiday then a change in eating habits (alcohol?) may be responsible. Are you unwell in crowded places, or in shops? If in shops, is it all shops or just one kind? These are often signs of chemical sensitivity. Fig 8 gives some of the allergens you should suspect if you have noticed any of these.

Next, think back over your life. Were you a colicky bottle-fed baby? Did you have food-fads as a child, or persistent constipation? Did you suffer from repeated throat infections or glue-ear? If so, you were probably food-sensitive as a child and food sensitivity may be surfacing again. Did your symptoms start after you moved home, or changed your eating habits, or your workplace? Often such associations are clear, the symptoms occurring quite soon

Fig 8   Some of the deductions to be drawn from variations in symptoms.

Deduction about the cause if:		
	Symptoms better	**Symptoms worse**
Times and Seasons		
At night		Mites, bedroom carpet, feathers, etc., moulds, ducted air, poor ventilation, pets
Morning		Mites, bedding, etc.
Mid-morning		Breakfast, newspapers, chemicals at work,
Evening		Food
Later in week		Chemicals at work
Weekend	Chemicals at work	Food (cycling, *see* Chapter 2)
Winter	Pollens	Inhalants, chemicals, heating

Outdoors		
Feb/May		Tree pollens
May/July		Grass pollens
May/Nov		Seasonal moulds
Places		
Heavy traffic		Petrol and diesel exhausts
Supermarkets, department stores		Chemicals, cigarette smoke, perfumes, air conditioning
Seaside	Pollens, moulds, chemicals	Pets (own or other peoples)
Country	Chemicals, vehicle exhausts	Pollens
Mediterranean, etc.	Mites, moulds, chemicals	Foods, local pollens
Skiing	Moulds	
Altitude	Mites	
Some houses		Moulds, gas, mites, chemicals, animals
Activities		
Exercise (asthma)		House dust, pets
Grass-cutting		Grass sap, pollen
Hedge-trimming		Privet sap
Vacuuming		Mites, animal dander, moulds
Cooking		Gas, moulds in kitchen
Alterations, DIY, etc.		Chemicals, dusts
Gardening	Chemicals, dusts in house	Pollens, moulds, sprays
Knitting		Wool (sheep, rabbit, etc.)
Missing meals		Foods, chemicals
Back home or to work after holiday		Mites, moulds, gas, etc. in house, chemicals, smoking etc. at work

after the change, but the interval between the two is sometimes long enough to make it difficult to recognise. If the change followed a move was it associated with the house itself, or its situation, or with a change in habits, or of food, associated with the move?

Lastly, think about your eating habits. Do you develop symptoms if you miss or delay a meal? If so, you are probably allergic to a very common food or foods. Have you tried conscientiously to lose weight and failed repeatedly? That is another characteristic finding in people who are food-allergic. Are there foods that you crave, or foods that you eat very frequently? If so, suspect these foods first. Did your symptoms start when you began to take some medication? Remember that reactions to drugs are not uncommon and can take many forms. Write all this information down and assess it – does it give you any pointers?

It is most unlikely that Type B reacters will have identified their allergens as a result of this exercise, but it may have given you a clue as to where to start. If you think food may be responsible, start with that. You will find details of how to set about it in Chapter 8. At the same time, start to take sensible precautions about the amount of chemical load to which you are exposed (*see* Chapter 6).

If you suspect that you are chemically sensitive, start by testing the substances whose smell you dislike (they are the most likely culprits), then test any others that could possibly be involved. Remember that if you are sensitive to one chemical, you are quite likely to be sensitive to others as well. First, try to avoid the chemical you want to test for a few days, a week if you can, but probably no longer. Then use the sniff test (*see* Chapter 1). Sit down in a comfortable chair and take the lid off the container holding the chemical (or piece of carpet or whatever) to be tested. Take a good sniff; stay sitting down quietly and then note whether you get any symptoms. If you are doubtful about your symptoms after 10 minutes take a few more good sniffs. Any chemical that causes symptoms should be avoided as far as possible in the future.

If you think that house dust mite is the major allergen, start by cleaning up your bedroom (*see* Chapter 6). That alone may make a substantial difference. If the problem is mould, deal with that. If you think you are sensitive to an animal kept in the house, you may be able to test this by going to stay in an animal-free house, having first washed all the clothes you plan to take. But remember, if the animal usually rides in the car with you, you will need to keep away from the car as well as the house while you are testing. In the case of pollen you can try staying indoors with the windows closed on a day with a high pollen count and see if your symptoms improve.

Sensitivity to these allergens can be confirmed by prick testing, which is routinely performed in conventional allergy clinics. However, it is as well to remember that although a positive test supports any observations you may have made indicating that the allergen is causing you problems, a negative test cannot *disprove* them. It is not unusual for prick tests to be negative when an allergen consistently causes symptoms.

Having improved while avoiding contact with an allergen, it is as well to test your conclusion by exposing yourself again to see what happens. The ideal time to challenge is between the fifth and fourteenth day since the last contact; this is when you get the clearest result. If you leave it longer than this you may need to test the substance several times over a few days before it is safe to assume that you are not going to react. Perfectionists would say that you should be tested in such a way that you do not know what is being tested: this is ideal, but usually impossible, and we find that open testing is quite satisfactory with nearly all patients. If you get symptoms on re-exposure you should avoid that contact in future, as far as this is possible.

In all your detective work you are looking for symptoms that are relieved by avoidance and then elicited by challenge with allergens. With some kinds of symptom it is a help to have a close relative or friend who will act as an observer. They will often notice if you *look* better more reliably than you can, and will be much better judges of irritability, unreasonableness and other mood changes, as well as being able to give more objective assessments. It is useful, too, to have their support and encouragement.

The central theme of this approach is to avoid those contacts that provoke symptoms, but remember to check with your doctor or a dietician before excluding foods in the longer term, to make sure that the remaining diet is nutritionally adequate; this is particularly important with children. There are two reasons for avoiding allergens to which you react: because the symptoms are disabling and unpleasant, and because reacting makes you more likely to develop further allergies. Avoiding reactions gives your immune system a chance to recuperate. Many people believe that recovery is more likely if chemical load can be reduced: there is no proof that this is so, but it seems probable, and a wise course to take while we wait for its full significance to be evaluated.

6
Practical Avoidance Measures

There are a wide variety of allergens to which you may react, and if you are to pin-point them, and institute successful avoidance measures, you need to be able to recognise the origin of those that may be involved, and know how to reduce exposure. First, you should look at your environment and decide which factors are most likely to cause your symptoms, and then proceed either to get rid of them or to reduce your exposure to a minimum.

INHALANTS

Moulds

Moulds occur everywhere, indoors and outdoors. Outdoors you can do little more than making sure that there are no unnecessary piles of leaves or of decaying vegetation near the house. If you are about to move, choosing the location of your new house is very important. Much higher concentrations of mould occur in low-lying areas, especially near still or running water; the presence of trees also encourages mould growth. So preferably choose a relatively open site, which is well drained and away from water.

Indoors, moulds grow in all sorts of places where you are not aware of them, encouraged by damp and poor ventilation. Firstly, go round the outside of the house to make sure all the ventilation bricks are unobstructed, and that soil and debris is not touching the wall higher than 6in (15cm) below the damp course. Then go right round your house inside and see if you can pick up any mouldy patches on the corners of walls (particularly outside walls), in bathrooms and kitchens (where most of the moisture is produced), under sinks, in cupboards, behind the back of cupboards, and so on. Moulds are especially likely to grow behind cupboards that are against outside walls, as the cupboard prevents the circulation of air and condensation occurs. Check for any damp anywhere; radiators that might be dripping on to carpets, leaking sinks or leaking piping, particularly where slight leaks might be concealed behind furniture or fittings. Any damp patch will grow moulds, and a surprisingly small area of damp will produce a vast number of mould spores, which can cause a lot of trouble to a mould-sensitive patient. Inspect windows and window frames carefully; even double-glazed windows collect enough condensation to encourage mould growth. Deal effectively with any leaks that you find, consult a good builder about any other damp patches, and check that there is good ventilation in any affected room. Damp mouldy patches should be treated by removing the source of damp and then treating with bleach before redecorating. There are some modern fungicides which are useful in some circumstances, but not recommended for anyone who may be chemically-sensitive. Putting a cup of bleach and vinegar (half and half) into a room and sealing the room for 24 hours is a useful way of killing growths of mould, and borax is also a good fungicide, particularly useful for those who cannot tolerate the others. It can be sprinkled in damp places and added (½ cup) to rinsing water to retard mould growth. Minimise mould round house plants by covering the soil with sand, and watering from the bottom.

Always check in wardrobes to make sure that there are no clothes or shoes at the back that have become mouldy. If they are needed and cannot be thrown away, mouldy clothes should be well washed and then thoroughly dried. Shoes should be dried and brushed well (by someone who is not mould-sensitive) and then put out in the sun to kill the mould. They should be inspected frequently to make sure the problem does not recur.

Humidity is a major cause of mould growth, so every allergic household should take general measures to try and reduce humidity in the house to a minimum. The major sources of humidity are the kitchen and the bathroom; both these areas should have extraction fans to reduce excess moisture, especially whilst anyone is cooking or having a bath or shower. Avoid drying clothes in the house, as far as possible, except in a tumble dryer vented to the outside. Any form of gas heater that releases heat into the house tends to release moisture as well, because water is formed when gas burns; the gas cooker is the worst offender but portable gas heaters are also bad; both produce excess condensation.

A good way of reducing the humidity level is to make sure that there is adequate ventilation throughout the house. This does not mean that there has to be a howling gale all day long, but it does mean that windows should be kept open slightly to make sure that there is a constant air exchange throughout the 24-hour period. Ordinary fireplaces are very good at improving circulation of air, as large amounts are sucked up the chimney when the fire is burning, and this ensures that fresh air is drawn in through the various windows and doors leading into the house. Ventilation is important in the bedroom at night, since every adult produces nearly a pint of water vapour in their breath and sweat in the course of each night.

Pollens

Wind-carried pollens are more difficult to avoid. Pollen counts are often given in the daily newspapers, or on the news, and on days when pollen is reported as high, or days that *you* recognise as producing high pollen counts, stay indoors, or stay inside the car with the windows closed as much as possible. It may help to have a recommended air filter in the house, but the advantage will only be felt if you are able to stay in that room. In the past, desensitisation has helped many of these patients; this is virtually unobtainable in the UK now, and the only constructive alternative is to seek out an allergist using the modern neutralisation technique (*see* Chapter 9). This can be effective in some cases.

The severely sensitive patient who has to go out will gain some advantage from fitting a filter in the car. Some cars have an air-cycling facility incorporated into the ventilation system which prevents outside air being brought into the car, so if you are buying a new car, keep this in mind. Air can only be recirculated for short periods, but it can be used to cover short journeys or short periods of gross pollution. Cars with air-conditioning are better, and can be adapted to take a charcoal filter to remove chemicals as well.

If you take holidays during the pollen season, choose a place or time when the pollen count will be low. If you go abroad, go where the pollen season is over or where you can holiday on the coast with an onshore wind. If you stay in the UK, try and make sure that you are on the coastline where the normal direction of wind is onshore – the west or south-west coast. An onshore wind is largely free of pollen and should give you a symptom-free holiday.

Animals or Birds

If you are very sensitive to animals it is essential to avoid having any animal or bird in the home. In extreme sensitivity they cannot even be kept in the vicinity of the house. Certain people react to horses when they are 50–100 yards downwind of a hunt, or when they go to a circus, even though they may be 20–30 yards away from the nearest animal. Patients who are mildly sensitive can keep animals which can live outside the house – long-haired dogs, rabbits, and so on – but the person who is sensitive to the animal should avoid contact and keep exposure generally to a minimum. Remember that small animals are just as dangerous in this respect as large animals. Gerbils and hamsters, which are often kept in the living room, are just as bad if not worse, than a dog living in the kitchen or outside. It is often forgotten that these small animals give rise to much allergenic material during a 24-hour period, all of which is released into the living room.

Animals leave large quantities of allergen behind them when they have been in contact with carpets, bedding or clothing. For instance, a cat may cause serious allergy problems if it sleeps on the child's bed during the day, even if it is absent during the night. For this reason, animals should be excluded totally from the living area of the house, if any members of the household are sensitive to them.

Another thing to remember is that if you are sensitive to one sort of furred animal, you are liable to become sensitive to another, so it is not wise to buy a different kind of animal in the hope that it will remain safe. It is quite common for people to become sensitive after 6 months or a year, by which time it has become extremely difficult to get rid of the animal, as you and other family members have become fond of it. It is better not to take the risk in the first place.

House Dust Mites

If you are sensitive to dust or mites, cut down the house dust mite population by reducing the warm humid areas in which they breed, such as bedding, carpets and household furniture. Avoid using the sort of materials in which the house dust mite grows well (feathers, flock, kapok, horsehair) and use materials they do not like – man-made fibre or foam rubber. The bedroom and the living room have the highest populations of mites.

It is most important to tackle the bedroom because you spend a third or more of your life there. First consider the bedding. The bed itself should be made of non-allergenic materials (wood or metal) with no covered or upholstered areas. If the bed has springs they should not be enclosed by a cotton cover of any sort. The mattress should be foam rubber, or cotton; generally it should not be inner-sprung, as most mattresses of this sort contain horsehair, or other substances in which mites thrive. Both the sheets and the blankets should be cotton and the eiderdown or duvet should be of man-made fibre. The pillow should also be filled with hollow-fibre, other man-made fibre, or 'Dunlopillo'. All the bedding should be cleaned regularly, and the blankets and duvet washed *at least* once every 2–3 months. Airing the bedding makes a big difference, as both sunlight and low humidity kill off the house dust mites.

The bedroom itself should be kept as clean and uncluttered as possible: the floor should be of lino, wood, or cork tiles. A carpet should not be used in the bedroom of a severely allergic patient as this provides a breeding ground for mites: the average carpet may contain between 1,000 and 10,000 mites per square metre. In addition, animal danders, food particles, and so on, tend to collect in carpets and can never be satisfactorily removed, whereas a polished floor can be kept very clean – it can also be very attractive, and if necessary, washable rugs can be used round the bed. Cupboards should be kept to a minimum, and only currently-used clothing kept in them: clothing that is out of season should be stored either in a chest of drawers that is kept closed, or preferably in another room and kept dry. Curtains should be made of light material and washed at least once every month.

Dusting should be done with a damp duster, which picks up the dust particles. The bedroom should be vacuumed very frequently, but one must remember that most vacuum cleaners are less than 100 per cent efficient as far as removing allergens is concerned. Vacuum cleaners vary in power, and in efficiency in picking up the dust, but more importantly the fine dust particles go straight through the bags and are then redistributed all over the bedroom. Indeed, if the vacuum cleaner is very powerful they may go all over the house. The particles that can pass through the vacuum cleaner bag include animal danders, house dust mite faecal pellets, and pollen grains. Recently a new vacuum cleaner has been introduced which takes out all dust particles down to 0.5μ in diameter (*see* Appendix II); this ensures the removal of almost all allergenic particles. One question that allergists have always asked patients suspected of being sensitive to house dust or house dust mite is whether they react with sneezing, wheezing and other symptoms when they are vacuuming. Those who are sensitive usually say 'Yes'. Anyone thinking about it would have realised that developing symptoms while vacuuming must have meant that the patient was exposed to excess allergen, and that a major source of this was the redistribution of allergens by the vacuum cleaner itself. Using the new vacuum cleaner described, patients who have previously reacted while vacuuming find that they can clean without any problems at all, which shows that the allergens are no longer being redistributed. People who have managed to avoid vacuuming to date now find that they can do it – which is not always popular!

House dust mites and animal danders are also present in the rest of the house, so an effective vacuum cleaner should be used throughout, and should be of significant benefit if used regularly. Remember that all furniture stuffed with horsehair or other organic materials presents a fertile source of house dust mite allergen, and if necessary should be changed for more modern furniture, often made of synthetic foam in which mites do not multiply. Another source, as far as children are concerned, is stuffed toys. If a stuffed teddy bear is filled with flock, or other natural materials, house dust mites may be present in vast numbers. All furry toys should be checked, and those that are found to be stuffed with natural fibres should be restuffed with man-made fibre, and washed regularly to remove the mites that remain. This is a source of house dust mite allergy that is often missed.

There are other measures that can be taken to reduce the house dust mite population. Recently a new paint has been introduced that kills mites, and there are several sprays available which can be sprayed on to bedding, furniture and carpets. However, these measures may cause problems in the chemically-sensitive patient, and so should be used with caution. The sprays produced so far only kill the mites themselves, and do nothing to reduce the vast amount of highly allergenic mite faecal pellets. These are very difficult to remove whatever method is used, and will continue to cause problems for many months, even if the mites have been eradicated. The newer products that are now being developed combine a mite-killing agent with a substance that destroys the allergenic particles. If this proves effective and non-toxic it will revolutionise the management of mite allergy.

CHEMICALS IN THE HOME

Large numbers of chemicals are routinely used in homes, offices, public and personal transport, and schools. The place that we have most control over is our own house. Anyone who shows any evidence of chemical sensitivity (and frankly, anyone else who is allergic to a significant degree) should seriously consider reducing the chemical contamination of their own home. We must remember that chemicals are not only toxic, but can also produce reactions in patients at very low concentrations without anyone being aware of it. Reducing the chemical load may help to prevent the development of further allergies, both to the chemicals themselves and to other allergens. When considering your own home, you have to work methodically through the various sources of chemical contamination that can occur. Whether you make changes in the house now or not, it is worth remembering what is recommended so that whenever equipment, fittings, or decorations have to be renewed, the replacements chosen are *better* for the allergy sufferers who live in the house, and not worse.

Structure of the House

The ideal house is a middle-aged one that has not had any recent decoration or refitting and is in a dry location, with a good damp-proof course, and central heating with radiators heated by a boiler in an outhouse or garage. Modern homes often use a lot of artificially-made substances, such as hardboard, plasterboard, insulation board, compressed materials for flooring and ceilings, and plastics, all of which outgas (that is, give off volatile chemicals) for a number of years, sometimes throughout their useful life. Allergic households should be particularly wary of refitting the kitchen or the bedroom with compressed boards which give off formaldehyde in significant amounts.

Decorating materials are a potent source of chemicals, especially paints and emulsions which are now made with the addition of numerous substances to produce better surface finishes. If you are going to decorate your house you should look for low-odour paints, or less chemically-contaminated paints and plain emulsions which do not contain extra chemicals; a number are now available. Papers should not be vinyl. Remember that most wallpaper paste contains fungicide; the addition of a tablespoon of borax to a pint of starch paste will help deter moulds.

Decorating should never be undertaken during the winter months, for two reasons: firstly, the lower temperatures will prolong the drying-out period (some paints take at least a year to dry out adequately); and secondly, no one will want all the windows open in the cold weather to allow adequate ventilation.

Furnishings

Modern furniture can be made very simply but increasing amounts of particle board are now being used, and most upholstered furniture now uses man-made fibre throughout, both in the coverings and the stuffing, and it can be a potent source of chemical contamination. Curtains should be of cotton, or at least of a material which does not smell of chemicals. The worst sort of furnishings in the home as far as chemicals are concerned are modern carpets. Most carpets are now treated to be moth-proof, stain-proof, moisture-proof, and end up by being virtually 'human-proof'. Man-made fibre carpets can outgas for the duration of their life; wool carpets are much better, but, again, most are treated with chemicals. The only way to test carpets is to go round checking samples, and smelling them yourself, to see how much chemical you can detect. Ideally though, the very chemically-sensitive patient should avoid using new carpets.

Types of Heating

Ducted air heating is the worst system as dust and other particles are transported throughout the house, and if the air is heated by a gas boiler, some fumes may leak into the air and cause serious problems. The ideal form of heating is by radiators heated by any form of fuel, as long as the boiler is outside the house itself (preferably in a garage that does not have a communicating door to the house). Gas (from gas boilers, gas fires or gas cookers) causes reactions in a surprising number of people; even the fumes from a pilot light may be enough to cause symptoms in those who are very sensitive. Others may get reactions from fumes from oil-filled installations. Reactions to coal and wood fires are less common but do occur; electric fires are to be preferred. Electricity is best for cooking. Although microwave ovens are in many ways ideal for allergy patients, it has been alleged that they may cause ill effects; this awaits substantiation.

Other Factors

Insulation also contributes to indoor chemical pollution. Relatively recently it has been realised that urea formaldehyde foam (which has been used quite widely as a cavity wall insulation material) can result in quite high levels of formaldehyde being present in homes for some years after its installation. Fibreglass, which one would assume to be innocuous, can be coated with materials containing formaldehyde. Chemicals used for timber treatment are another problem; they can persist in the house for some considerable time after their application – houses that may require timber treatment in the future should be avoided.

DIY activities frequently involve the use of a number of chemicals. As far as possible, such activities should be done in the garage, or outside, and stringent care should be taken to ensure that frequent air changes are maintained throughout the time chemicals are in use and drying. Any other suggested precautions should also be strictly applied.

Newsprint, magazines and books all outgas, although some are worse than others. When you have noticed the smell of printed matter you will be surprised to what extent it contaminates the air in most houses. People who react to newsprint may find they can read without symptoms if the book, magazine or newspaper has been left in the oven overnight at the lowest setting, and then allowed to cool, or if it is put out in the sun for a time.

Chemicals used in Cleaning

You should reduce the numerous chemicals that are used in the house. Many cleaning products (including polishes, bleaches, soaps, detergents, and so on) now contain many extra chemicals, but some simple products are still obtainable and a number of hypo-allergic alternatives are on sale. Simple alternatives include the use of washing soda for heavy cleaning, bicarbonate of soda for washing floors, refrigerators, and so on (1 tbs/bucket), and clothes (2–3 tbs per wash load), vinegar for washing windows and baths, neat cider vinegar for polished chrome, a strong solution of bicarbonate of soda for silver, and table salt dampened with vinegar or lemon juice for brass, bronze and copper. Aerosols should be avoided because they are toxic and the aerosol droplets are very small and readily inhaled. There are also a large number of preparations on the market designed to make the house and the washing smell 'nice' – air-fresheners, deodorisers and clothing conditioners. These can all have disastrous effects on individuals who are sensitive to them, and are quite unnecessary. We have been brainwashed into thinking that ordinary human smells are unpleasant, but this is not so. Moreover, clothes used to smell and feel nice because they were dried in the fresh air, and this is still possible for many people (although not wise for the pollen-sensitive when pollen counts are high). The addition of borax to rinsing water helps to remove soap and odours.

Clothes that have been dry-cleaned smell strongly of the solvents used for several days, sometimes longer. They should never be put away in the bedroom until the smell has gone, and preferably they should not even be brought into the house in this condition, but hung up in the sun to speed up the drying-out process.

Personal Chemicals

The next group to consider comprises the various substances people use on themselves – perfumes, cosmetics of all sorts, body lotions, hair sprays, shampoos and soaps. The more the product smells, the more likely it is to be a risk. Women used to be the major offenders as far as toiletries were concerned, but recently men are using numerous highly-scented preparations. This has almost become a cult, but people who stop using them find they get much more enjoyment from natural smells. Alternatives to nearly all these substances are available in the shops, either hypo-allergenic and non-scented, or with a minimum of smell.

Another substantial source of chemicals is toothpaste, which often contains ten or more chemicals. A mixture of two parts of sea salt to one part of sodium bicarbonate, ground together, makes a satisfactory alternative which avoids the potentially harmful chemicals entirely. It is best to use this mixture while you are sorting out your problems, as some people have reactions to some of the chemicals in toothpaste. Later you could try one of the hypo-allergenic toothpastes free of additives (*see* Appendix II).

Lastly, cigarette smoke: many allergy sufferers find that cigarette smoke causes symptoms, or makes symptoms worse. Allergy sufferers should not smoke and should avoid other people's smoke as far as possible. Make your house and car a smoke-free zone – other people should respect your wishes.

CHEMICALS IN THE OFFICE

It is only recently that offices have become sealed and fully air-conditioned. Previously it was possible to open a window and let in fresh air, and even if the air was not very fresh in the centres of towns or cities, at least air circulation was provided and indoor pollutants had a chance to escape. Nowadays most buildings have windows that cannot be opened, and rely on air-conditioning systems which recycle the majority of air in the building, usually with only a simple fibre dust filter. Any chemicals released into the atmosphere by office processing machines, any chemicals worn by the people in the office, plus cigarette smoke, are simply recycled, creating a very unhealthy atmosphere. It is difficult to control the office environment, however, efforts can be made to reduce the amount of smoking, and people may perhaps be encouraged to wear less perfume. Fortunately, it is becoming more acceptable to provide a smoke-free area, and before long it is likely to become a legal requirement.

The chemicals present in other workplaces are outside the scope of this book. The workforce will usually be aware of them. These chemicals may also affect the families of workers (if taken home on the skin or clothes), and other people living in the vicinity.

CHEMICALS IN SCHOOLS

Modern schools are often chemically polluted to a serious extent. Old schools tend to be very dusty, but very few chemicals were used in their construction or in their furnishings. New schools are absolutely riddled with chemicals, in the structure, flooring and desks, as well as in the cleaning materials used, and the materials used in craft rooms and laboratories. Any non-smoker walking into a modern school will be very aware of how strong the chemical smell is throughout the buildings. This is a very difficult problem to solve. Schools should be given every encouragement to reduce the chemicals used or to change to products with little smell. There are now plenty of relatively non-allergenic products available which are the same price (or minimally more expensive) than the products in use, and there is no reason why they should not be adopted universally. However, pressure from the parents will be needed before anything changes. In view of the fact that symptoms from chemicals commonly include panic attacks, mood changes (including aggression), and difficulties with writing or spelling, it would be wise for *all* parents to bring their influence to bear on this issue, whether their own child is affected or not. Adequate ventilation in classrooms is also imperative.

CHEMICALS IN PUBLIC PLACES

We have seen a very healthy change in the attitude towards

smoking in the last 10 years. Until recently there was no restriction on smoking in public places, but this has now changed and it is to be hoped that this trend will continue. Ideally, all public places (except open space) should totally ban smoking, and this includes theatres, cinemas and restaurants, and all public transport, on land, sea and in the air. We are beginning to see this in the USA and UK where some airlines are banning smoking on shorter flights: hopefully this will gradually be extended.

Most large stores have restricted ventilation systems, frequently inadequate for removing chemicals given off by the goods, the staff and the clients: contamination is particularly bad in areas selling perfumery, plastics, plastic-wrapped goods and carpets.

CHEMICALS IN FOOD AND WATER

Most people who are food-allergic react to the foodstuffs themselves, and here the major part of management is identification of the food and subsequent careful avoidance. Food additives (and sometimes contaminents) also need to be tested, and if necessary avoided in the same way (Chapter 8).

Adulteration and contamination of food and water with chemicals was considered in Chapter 3. What can we, as individuals, do to reduce the chemicals we absorb in food? The main thing is to eat mainly freshly-prepared food, with a minimum of junk food, reading labels carefully to choose varieties with the least additives, and avoiding any food where sugar and fats are listed unexpectedly early in the list of ingredients. The predominance of these foodstuffs usually needs to be disguised with dyes and artificial flavours. Chemicals from soft plastic migrate into food, particularly into fat left in contact with the plastic for long periods. Food that has been wrapped in plastic should be unwrapped and left to air for some hours before use, to allow the chemicals to diffuse. It is preferable to use cellophane for wrapping food (for advice, *see* Appendix II). Aluminium pans should be replaced – aluminium from pans contaminates food cooked in them, particularly acid foods, and any other type of pan is preferable. Many people already use sea salt or pure salt to avoid the additives in table salt, and organic produce when it is available.

Practical Avoidance Measures

We should all make sure that informed public pressure is kept up promoting the reduction of additives in food, in the use of pesticides and herbicides, and in the release of chemicals into the environment. We can press for measures to encourage organic growers, and continue to encourage them with our custom.

What practical steps can we take about water contamination since we are all dependent on the water supplied to us? There are quite a large number of water filters appearing on the market. The active constituent in the majority of these is activated charcoal, and an adequate amount of this substance will remove most of the common chemicals that are in the water supply. However, nitrates are not removed by this process, and are generally much more difficult to tackle. There are now several filters available which can remove nitrates, most using reverse osmosis, but these tend to be expensive both to buy and to run. It is likely that better and cheaper filters will be developed and eventually most private households will have their own filter for drinking water. The alternative to using a filter is to buy one of the numerous types of bottled spring water that are now available in all supermarkets and health food stores. Most of these waters are tested and are reasonably pure, although this is an area that is open to abuse and which needs to be watched carefully. Many are bottled in plastic which can cause problems for some people. Each person needs to test their chosen water.

By being aware of what is added to foods, reading the books describing the use of the various additives and the limitations of labelling, reading labels carefully, choosing foods and water wisely, and favouring organic farming, everyone can reduce their consumption of chemicals to a minimum. However, it is imposs-ible to eliminate them completely, even if you grow all your own food without chemicals and away from roads. This is the price we have to pay for our lifestyle and for modern food production, but it need not be as bad as it is. Intake is higher in the UK than in many other countries because of the permissive attitude that has been adopted towards food additives, an addiction to junk foods and the high concentration of population. For the future of the country, changes are needed quickly.

7

The Ideal House for Allergics

This chapter is for those who plan to build a house, or to alter their present home. We shall bring together advice on building and equipping a house which could be passed on to your architect or builder so that they understand what you want. It is based on experience gained with the Airedale Allergy Centre, an environmentally-controlled in-patient unit built to exclude chemicals and inhalants as much as is possible. The core of the construction information was obtained from Dr Randolph in Chicago and Dr Rea in Dallas, who first developed such units, in which even the most severely ill environmental patients will clear. Less rigorous alternatives are also given since most allergy patients do not need such a controlled environment. However, anyone from an allergic family would be wise to take some precautions when building or converting a house; it might prevent a marked deterioration in their symptoms.

IDEAL SITUATION

When selecting a suitable site, compromises are inevitable. As far as possible, avoid situations exposed to heavy traffic fumes, but also avoid being closely surrounded by woods, or by farmland which is likely to carry hay crops or to be sprayed regularly. Avoid a site in a hollow where moulds and atmospheric pollution collect when there is no wind, sites near water of any sort as this encourages moulds, and those downwind (even several miles away) of industry. In the UK most allergy patients feel best at the seaside, particularly on the west coast with the prevailing wind coming off the sea.

STRUCTURE

The house may be built of stone, brick or concrete (provided that no chemical accelerators or retardants were added to the concrete). Avoid houses with a large amount of wood, as chemicals used to treat wood may outgas for years. Make sure there is a good damp-proof course, and that water and soil are kept away from the walls. Avoid any house that needs a new damp-proof course or one that needs preservative treatment to woodwork. Avoid over-exposure to dust in the course of alterations; do not be afraid to use a mask whenever you have to be near dust.

The plan of the house may be conventional except that the boiler for the central heating should be in an outhouse or garage without direct access to the house, preferably downwind of the house and with a chimney high enough to ensure that fumes do not enter the house even when the wind is contrary. If this is followed, any type of fuel can be used. Ducted air central heating should *not* be installed. Water circulation systems are satisfactory, while under-floor electric heating is less good and usually expensive to run. Oil-filled electric radiators offer an alternative, and electric fires with the element embedded in ceramic are satisfactory, but fan heaters and some types of night storage heaters can be troublesome. In a new house solar panels might be worth considering, even though some form of back-up heating would be needed. Many allergic people cannot tolerate an open fire, although for those who can, open fires have the advantage of improving ventilation. Avoid gas fires, and gas back-boilers.

Kitchen and bathrooms should have extract fans, and airbricks. Care should be taken in siting these to ensure that the air-flow crosses the source of moisture and of smells, so that these are cleared when the fan is running. Bathrooms should be adequately heated and have plenty of towel rails so that towels can be spread out. Cooking should be by electricity. An extra cold tap should be installed in the kitchen to take a water filter. If a tumble dryer is used it should be vented to the outside; if not, provision should be made for washing to be dried in an outhouse or carport in bad weather. Ideally the washer and dryer should be in a separate well-ventilated room, and possibly the freezer should be as well.

Whether the boiler is in the garage or not, there should *not* be direct access from the garage to the house. Isolated outside storage for things not tolerated in the house can be useful. The provision of ventilation in the frames of windows is valuable: good ventilation is *essential*. Bedrooms should be kept bare and simple; fitments should be made of real wood, and the provision of a small, warm and well-ventilated dressing-room would be ideal, so that clothes need not be kept in the bedroom.

The environmental unit has a ducted positive-pressure ventilation system with a bank of filters to exclude particles down to 0.5μ and to absorb chemicals. Similar systems can be obtained for houses but would be rather expensive. Severely allergic people may otherwise find they have to make themselves a safe oasis within the house, in which the air is continuously filtered using a portable air filter, spending either their nights, or even most of their time in that room. Few people are as sensitive as this.

MATERIALS

Avoid the use of compressed boards of all kinds as the glue which sticks the particles together outgasses for several years. This includes all boards made by glueing, insulation boards, and compressed boarding for floors, furnishings and fittings, and hardboard. Kitchen units should be of stainless steel, or of wood which could be surfaced with formica or similar, provided you do not react to the adhesive used to fix it. Working tops could be of stainless steel or of tiles on a wooden base.

Use rockwool or fibreglass for insulating the walls, asking for a type that is *not* chemically treated. Use untreated fibreglass for the roof space. Window frames should be of hardwood or aluminium. The woodwork should be of real wood throughout, preferably hardwood in the living space. Outside, the wood can be treated with linseed oil, while inside it can be polished with basic wax polish or sealed with several coats of polyurethane varnish. Polyurethane is satisfactory in the longer term as it dries quickly and has stopped outgassing by about three months, but care should be taken to keep away from newly-treated woodwork. The floors should be of hardwood, sealed in the same way, or be covered with ceramic tiles or cork tiles which can also be sealed. Avoid carpets as far as possible, particularly in the bedroom. Washable rugs are satisfactory, provided they are washed regularly

If you have been able to use hardwood, little or no paint will be necessary. If this has not been possible, use a low-odour paint and ventilate well. Plain emulsions that have minimal additional chemicals are all right for many people. You should avoid vinyl wallcoverings, but paper wallpapers are satisfactory if stuck on with a safe paste. Avoid products treated with fungicide. Avoid all soft plastic fittings (lampshades, hangings, and so on); most people have no trouble with fittings made of hard plastic.

FURNISHINGS

Avoid soft plastics in any form. Avoid horizontal venetian blinds (which collect dust) unless you are prepared to be meticulous about damp-dusting, at least weekly. If you use carpets in any rooms, choose those with as little chemical smell as possible. Artificial fabrics outgas, and most wool carpets are treated with moth-proofing and stain-resisting agents. Curtains and rugs should be readily washable (particularly in the bedroom), preferably of cotton, but certainly avoiding materials smelling of chemicals. Upholstery should *not* be of feather or horsehair. Most people can manage latex foam or man-made fibre, but try smelling it first. Some quite comfortable cane furniture is available. Much modern furniture is made of compressed boards which may outgas for years. Older furniture of real wood is preferred, but if it is very old be sure to smell it to make sure that it has not been chemically treated recently. Give it a good scrub, particularly in the drawers and in other places where dust and mould accumulate, then dry and air it well afterwards. Most people can tolerate a latex foam mattress for the bed; this should be on a simple base, either wooden with ventilation holes, or of exposed springs. Avoid conventional upholstered springing for bed or mattress, and avoid dust traps anywhere. The most allergen-free beds are those with metal frames, simple open springing and cotton mattresses. More comfortable all-cotton interior-sprung mattresses are also available (*see* Appendix II for advice), and are perfectly acceptable, provided that they are regularly vacuumed for dust and mites.

8
Exclusion Diets

A number of principles concerning exclusion diets have been worked out over the last sixty years: before embarking on such a diet it is important to understand these principles, otherwise it can be very confusing and even dangerous. The stricter exclusion diets should be used only under medical or dietary supervision. If strict diets go on for too long, nutritional deficiencies may occur and compound the whole problem; this is a particular risk with young children. In this chapter we concentrate on the simpler exclusion diets which you can do on your own.

PRINCIPLES OF EXCLUSION DIETS

Exclusion diets rely on the finding that if you exclude a food from your diet for an adequate time, and then eat it as a 'challenge', any reaction to it will be more obvious than when you are eating it continuously. It will then be clear to you from your reactions which foods are safe and which are causing problems. It is important that the exclusion of the food is *total*: if even the tiniest amount of food you have been reacting to remains in your diet, it may invalidate the challenge phase of the diet. This may be quite difficult to achieve. Modern eating habits have changed markedly over the last forty years. Foods used to be simple and contain few ingredients. Since the 1940s more and more food mixtures have come into use, and certain foodstuffs are now included in a number of different items that are eaten every day (Fig 9). Soya and corn are good examples. Thirty years ago soya was infrequently used in the UK, although widely used in the USA, but its use has increased dramatically. Its main forms are soya oil, soya flour, soya beans and textured soya protein (TSP). It is used in pre-prepared and pre-packaged meat products, is present in nearly all bread, appears in many vegetable oils, and is the oil most often used in cans of fish such as pilchards; it also occurs in many other foods.

Fig 9   Some hidden sources of common foods.

Yeast	Vinegar – dressings, mayonnaise, sauces, pickles; all alcohol and alcoholic beverages, malt; fruit juices, tinned or frozen; bread and breadcrumbs, etc.; cheeses (all kinds); mushrooms, surfaces of root vegetables; antibiotics, vitamin B; Marmite, Yeastvite.
Milk	*Look for whey, lactose, casein, lactalbumin, milk solids, milk fats.* Butter, cheese, yoghurt, cream, curds; most margarines (*not* Tomor, Vitaquel, Vitasig, Granose or FoodWatch); cakes, pancakes, batters, some pastry, some breads and rolls; glazing on bread, biscuits; scrambled egg, omelette, egg custard; ice cream, milk chocolate and some others, toffee, some sweets; butter, and anything cooked in it; cream soups, sometimes other soups, meat products, etc.; mashed potato, foods 'au gratin'; all white sauces, butter sauces, salad dressing.
Egg	Mayonnaise, salad cream, tartare sauce; cakes, fritters, batters, pancakes; glazing on bread, biscuits; pasta; meringues, sponge puddings, custards; some sauces, soups, biscuits; wine, beer.
Corn	Corn oil, vegetable oil, margarines, ice cream, crisps; cornflour (used for thickening), soups, gravies; glucose, dextrose; corn syrup (most sweets and soft drinks and many alcoholic drinks); gums (stamps, envelopes), some coffee substitutes.
Soya	Soya oil, vegetable oil; soya protein (TSP, in many made-up dishes to extend meat); soya milk; soya flour (most breads).
Wheat	Bread, biscuits, cakes, pastries, batters; pasta, some poppadoms, noodles; sausages, canned meats, soups, gravy; anything in breadcrumbs; some salad dressings, some ice creams; some coffee substitutes, some whisky, some malt; many tinned foods, most pre-prepared foods; puddings, pies, stuffings; most sauces.

When you are thinking about following an exclusion diet you have to go back to basics. Look at all the foods you normally eat and break them down as far as you can into the individual ingredients: you may have some surprises. In fact, the only satisfactory way of doing an exclusion diet is to leave out pre-prepared and pre-packaged foods entirely; there is no other way of being certain that you have excluded all the foods you are trying to avoid. Throughout the diet it is essential to be absolutely thorough in your approach, so make detailed plans before starting.

THE DURATION OF THE EXCLUSION PHASE

Different people recommend different durations for the exclusion phase of the diet. The principle is that you should exclude the foods until they are out of your system completely. The time varies in different people, largely depending on how long it takes for food to be eliminated from the body – the bowel transit time. Ideally, this should be 24 hours or less, but in Western society constipation is very common, and occasionally patients may even be constipated for as long as 6 to 8 weeks (although this is exceptional). In these cases the body would not be clear of the food eaten for about the same length of time, as residual food may be absorbed from the large bowel. Take a mild aperient at the beginning of the elimination diet, to clear your system, and then 5 to 10 days will probably be adequate. If your symptoms are continuing to improve, avoid re-introducing the food (or any of the foods) until your symptoms have stabilised for several days.

THE FOOD CHALLENGE STAGE

You are then ready to start food challenges. A single food or drink should be re-introduced first thing in the morning. Food can be tested at other times of the day, but you get a clearer result if you have not eaten for about 12 hours, and first thing in the morning is the only time you can guarantee this. If you normally eat a snack late at night be sure to avoid having anything except water from 8p.m. the night before testing.

How much should you take to produce a conclusive result? That depends on how sensitive you think you are. If you suspect that you are very sensitive to that food, start with a very small amount and then take more if you have not reacted – a mouthful or two first thing, twice as much half an hour later if nothing has happened, and a normal-sized portion if nothing has happened after an hour. For example, with coffee: at 7.30a.m. have literally 2 or 3 tea-spoonsfuls of a cup of black unsweetened coffee; at 8a.m. try a quarter of a cupful; at 8.30a.m. if you are still symptom-free take at least one cupful of strong coffee, if not two, again black and unsweetened, and await the results. If you have no reason to suppose that you are particularly sensitive to the food you are going to test, there is no need to take these precautions; just take a normal helping on the first occasion. If in the past you have ever had a severe reaction to any food, do not embark on *any* testing without a doctor's advice and supervision.

REACTIONS

How quickly should you expect to have a reaction? In Type A allergy reactions are immediate. They can start within 30 seconds to a minute and be at their maximum within 4 minutes; they rarely start later than a quarter to half an hour after ingestion, and do not normally last longer than 1 to 2 hours. In Type B allergy, the picture is quite different. Although they may start relatively quickly, the majority of reactions are slower, coming on at some time within the first 4 hours. It is possible for the onset of some reactions to be delayed longer, occasionally for 24 hours or more.

A number of factors contribute to the variation, including individual differences. A major factor is the nature of the food and how it is prepared. If the food is a simple foodstuff such as coffee or tea, or especially alcohol, reactions tend to be quick. With more complex foods such as wheat (or one of the other grains), reactions are usually delayed and occasionally will not start for 2 or 3 days, even if the person eats the food 3 times a day.

The length of time the person has avoided that food also affects the speed of onset, because tolerance may start to develop after a gap of 3 weeks or so. To illustrate this, let us look at the coffee-drinker again, someone who is getting symptoms from drinking 6 cups of coffee a day. If they stop drinking coffee, 5 or 6 days later their symptoms clear. In the next few days, testing will give an acute reaction that comes on fairly rapidly. If they wait a month they only get a mild reaction after one cup of coffee or no reaction at all, but if they drink 3 to 4 cups of coffee a day they will soon start to feel ill, and the reaction will gradually build up. If they wait 3 months, it may take a week or 2 weeks for the first symptoms to appear, even if they are consuming 3 or 4 cups a day. If they wait a year, they may have become fully tolerant and be able to drink coffee in moderation from then on without getting any symptoms. However, the majority of patients with Type B symptoms find that if they go back to their old habits, and consume the food as often as they did originally, their tolerance eventually breaks down, and they become sensitive again.

There are, therefore, two basic things you must remember. You must not be off the food too long, or else tolerance may occur and a reaction will be missed, and you must not be off the food for too short a time, or else the body may not be clear of that food and again reactions may be missed.

MASKING

This brings us to the concept of masking, which is another very important aspect that must be understood before attempting any testing. Masking refers to the state of the patient who is consuming a food so frequently that he is totally unaware that it upsets him. He has chronic symptoms but he cannot correlate any of them with the foods he is consuming.

Again, take the coffee-drinker who drinks 6 to 8 cups a day as an example. If the reaction comes on quickly and is very short he will know that after each cup he becomes unwell, and that he is back to normal before he has the next cup. But if the reaction takes several hours to come on and can last up to 24 hours, then it is easy to see that the reaction from the first cup of coffee in the morning may not have reached its peak by the time the second cup is taken, so the symptoms will build up during the day. If he consumes his last cup of coffee last thing at night, or if his reaction time is rather long, his symptoms may not even have improved before he has a cup of coffee next morning. This is masking, and once it has occurred the fluctuation of symptoms during the day, or from day to day, may be minimal.

Masking does not usually occur with foods eaten less frequently than every 4 days, but can with foods eaten more often than that, especially if they cause long-lasting, or delayed symptoms. So when you are doing any sort of exclusion diet the absolute minimum time to avoid the food before testing is 4 days; anything less than this may result in a reaction being missed.

FOOD ADDICTION

Addiction to foods occurs frequently, and behaves in much the same way as any other addiction. It is closely related to masking. When patients have masked reactions to a food they may have almost constant symptoms (or intermittent 'cycling' symptoms) which actually get better immediately after eating that particular food. They experience a transient 'high' just as drug addicts do, but this lasts only a short time, and afterwards they feel worse. They do not realise the food is causing the symptoms, so they eat it more and more frequently and become worse and worse. Only when the addiction is broken by avoiding the food for at least 4 or 5 days does the true nature of the relationship become apparent.

CHOICE OF FOODS TO TEST

If you suspect that you have a food allergy, which foods should you choose to test? The first ones to suspect are those you consume most frequently. A simple way of finding these is to keep a food diary for a week. Simply write down everything you eat or drink for 7 days; this must include all drinks, all sweets and chewing gum, and even drugs, as these contain other ingredients (including actual foodstuffs such as cornflour and potato starch), and if you are on regular medication this may need to be taken into account when you are assessing what you eat; at present this is difficult, but details about the contents of all medicines will soon be made available to doctors and pharmacists, who will then be able to pass the information on to you.

At the end of the week you should add up the number of times you have eaten each individual food. To do this you need to break down any pre-prepared food into the individual ingredients. For instance, at breakfast you have toast, margarine, marmalade and coffee with milk and sugar. What have you actually eaten? Firstly you have obviously had coffee, milk and sugar once. What is in margarine? It contains numerous ingredients including colourings, flavourings, preservatives and anti-oxidants, certain oils (such as soya oil, sunflower seed oil and/or others), and often milk solids in the form of whey, casein or lactose. What is in the bread? Bread contains wheat and yeast, probably soya, a small amount of sugar and an oil of some sort, in addition to any of about 48 substances that can be added to flour. The marmalade? That obviously contains sugar (or maybe corn as corn syrup) and oranges, but it may also contain such things as saccharine, gelatine, or other additives. So at breakfast you may have consumed more than twenty different substances.

You need to do this with all the foods you eat during the week, and then add up the total number of times you have eaten each individual food. You are most likely to be reacting to the foods that come at the top of the list. There is a clear correlation between the frequency of eating a certain foodstuff and the likelihood of becoming allergic to it, although the reason for this is not known. The foods you pick out to test should therefore be the ones you consume most frequently; normally these are wheat, corn (maize), dairy products, sugar, tea, coffee and eggs. You may have a considerable surprise when you break down your diet; you may have thought that you did not eat the same foods very often, but you will find that certain foods come up again and again. Remember that if you drink a cup of tea 10 times a day with milk and sugar in, that is 10 times for milk, sugar and tea, so don't cheat. The only person you will be cheating is yourself.

WITHDRAWAL

What can you expect to happen when you embark on an exclusion diet? Here again you may get some surprises. It is not nearly as simple as you might think. For a long time people running health farms have used diets to help people regain health, some clients even fasting for a short time, and it has been recognised that some people feel ill temporarily when they go on a strict diet. A perfectly healthy peson who has no evidence of food allergy or intolerance feels no ill effects if they fast. They develop no symptoms, except for hunger, and after 2 days the hunger settles and they feel well. If a person who suffers from significant food allergy goes on a diet to avoid the foods that upset them, they go through what is called a 'withdrawal reaction'. This can last for anything from 1 to 14 days (and very occasionally longer). The duration is usually related to the severity of the reaction to foods, and to the number of food sensitivities. However, if you are severely sensitive to one food, you may get a bad withdrawal reaction, which may even be worse than if you are mildly sensitive to a dozen foods. The severity also relates to how thorough you are with your diet. If you happen to succeed in removing all the foods to which you are sensitive, you will suffer from a much more severe withdrawal reaction than if you only remove half of those foods. So welcome the severity as evidence that you are on the right track. The withdrawal reaction usually starts within 18 hours of stopping the food concerned, but it can be delayed for 2 days or longer.

Some people notice that under ordinary circumstances they cannot miss, or even delay, a meal without becoming ill. These people are usually food-allergic and are suffering from a naturally-occurring withdrawal reaction.

During withdrawal you may suffer from all sorts of symptoms. There may be an exaggeration of your normal symptoms, possibly to the extent of giving you the most severe attack you have had for a long time. A typical example is migraine. Someone who suffers from migraine, perhaps every fortnight, may get the worst migraine he has had for months when he goes on an exclusion diet. This may start by about 1p.m. on the day he started avoiding the food; it peaks the following day, and clears during the third or fourth day. In addition, there are a number of other symptoms which may occur. The most common is a diffuse aching in the bottom, thighs or legs, which characteristically starts on about the second day, lasts 3 or 4 days, and can be severe enough to keep the sufferer awake for 2 or 3 nights. Other symptoms are either sleepiness or insomnia, fatigue, restlessness, aching joints, skin rashes, sweating and shivering.

Sometimes the symptoms are so severe that the patient may think he is dying by about the second day, but there has never been a recorded death during an exclusion diet. You may feel awful but it is not actually harming you: the worst withdrawals may mimic the reaction experienced by a heroin addict when he stops heroin, but it will not be quite as severe. Pain-killers can be used, but are often surprisingly ineffective. At this stage it is important to persevere, whether you feel like it or not. If you give way and have your favourite food all your symptoms may clear in 10 to 15 minutes. You will have had your 'shot' and will be temporarily better, but the symptoms will soon be back in the same intractable form as before. If you can manage to keep going, by about the fourth day your symptoms will start to clear, and by the sixth to eighth day you will feel marvellous. All the symptoms will have gone, and you will feel on top of the world – often better than you have for years.

When you feel clear like this, it is time to start re-introducing the foods you want to test. Always allow yourself a day or so of feeling well before attempting to make yourself ill again by testing foods, especially if you have suffered from a bad withdrawal reaction. Sort out which foods you want to test. The speed of re-introduction again varies from person to person and from diet to diet. If you are doing an exclusion diet at home, then simply re-introduce one food a day, taking the food first on its own at breakfast-time, and repeating it at lunch-time and tea-time if you get no reaction. If you still feel well the next day you can be reasonably confident that you do not react to that food. However, if you have been off the food for longer than a month, it is important to take the food for several days running before assuming that it does not upset you, in case tolerance has started to develop. This is why we tend to use short-duration diets, and fairly rapid re-introduction, which largely avoids the errors that can arise from partial tolerance.

SYMPTOMS AND SIGNS OF REACTIONS

What do you look for when re-introducing food? First, look for a recurrence of the symptoms from which you were suffering, especially those you have had for a very long time. Don't ignore any symptoms that occur, because even if you have taken them for granted for years, they may disappear on exclusion, and suddenly reappear on food challenge. Fig 2 will remind you about the wide range of symptoms that may be involved.

When you are doing challenges it is often useful to ask someone else who knows you well to help. The reason for this is that they may notice changes in you that you either do not notice, or ignore, thinking that they are normal. This is particularly the case with mood changes. These are quite commonly caused by food reactions and are usually unrecognised by the person concerned. However, the rest of the family (who suffer from them indirectly) will recognise them much more easily, so a wife, husband, boy-friend, girlfriend, and so on, can be a great help. As long as they understand the position, they can also give you encouragement and support, which can make a lot of difference.

In addition to recognising the specific reactions, it is important to monitor objective signs. First, look at your body weight. Quite a high proportion of people experience rapid body weight changes when they go on an exclusion diet and when they re-introduce some of the test foods. It has been shown repeatedly that those people who suddenly gain weight when they go away for the weekend, or out for an evening, are the ones who do the same while they are testing foods, after eating only a small amount of a food to which they react. It is important to weigh yourself accurately night and morning, and to record your weight, as you carry out the food challenges. A gain in weight of more than 1lb (1/2kg) suggests that a food has upset you; a gain in weight of several pounds after eating a certain food is strong evidence that the food is bad for you, even in the absence of any other signs or symptoms.

The second method of observation was described originally by Dr Coca in the USA, and is called the *pulse test*. Nearly everyone is capable of taking their own pulse; if you do not know how to do it, ask someone who is medically trained to show you. You need to take a *resting* pulse rate so each time before taking it sit down for 5 minutes resting, then count the beats for 30 seconds (or for a full minute). (If you count for half a minute simply multiply the figure by 2 to get your minute pulse rate.) You should practise this before you go on the exclusion diet, so that you know how to get an accurate reading. Take your pulse before you eat the food and 20,

40 and 60 minutes afterwards. Make out a special chart using the same columns as in the one on page 107, and write down the readings as you go along, or you will forget them. A pulse change, either up or down, of more than 10 beats per minute is significant, and usually means that the food has upset you, even in the absence of other symptoms and signs.

About two-thirds of the population are 'pulse responders', in other words, people who get pulse changes after eating certain foods. The other third show no change at all. The same thing applies to weight: only a proportion of people respond with a weight gain after eating certain foods. By observing weight, pulse and symptoms you can recognise the foods that upset you fairly accurately.

In the course of your investigation you may find that your pulse rate gradually settles to a lower resting level. This happens quite frequently and shows that the previous resting level was raised by chronic reactions. Doctors working in this field have also noticed that patients with raised blood pressure experience a fall in blood pressure when foods they were reacting to are withdrawn, and may use this as an additional sign. Dizziness occuring during an exclusion diet should be reported to your doctor as it could be a result of a fall in blood pressure.

Once you are certain that you are reacting to a food, what can you do about stopping the full development of the reaction? A very simple way, described in the USA, is to take alkali salts, consisting of 2 parts sodium bicarbonate and 1 part potassium bicarbonate. In the USA it is sold as 'Alka Seltzer Gold', for indigestion. 'Alka Seltzer' in the UK consists of alkali and aspirin, so it is not a good idea to take it, especially if you are aspirin-sensitive. You should either take a dose of sodium bicarbonate on its own, or obtain the alkali mixture from your chemist, or by mail order (*see* Appendix II). One to two teaspoonfuls in half a tumbler of warm water can often settle food reactions quickly. Another good alkali mixture is one teaspoonful of powdered vitamin C (*see* Appendix II for source advice) with up to half a teaspoonful of sodium bicarbonate in water. If the mixture is correct, this is quite pleasant to take.

If you have had a reaction, you should wait until you feel well before going on to test the next food, rather than rushing on and testing it the next day. You will obtain a clearer result if you allow yourself time to recover fully. If you test a second food while you are still reacting to the first, you may get a false positive reaction, and if this happens with several consecutive foods the whole picture can become extremely confusing, and it may be quite impossible to interpret your results.

TYPE OF DIET

Excluding a Single Food

What sort of diet could you use? The simplest diet consists of excluding a single food such as tea, coffee or chocolate. Avoiding soya, egg, or milk is more complicated because they appear in so many other foods (Fig 9). If, for example, you think you are having far too much coffee, then stop drinking it altogether, also stop drinking tea, chocolate, Lucozade, and cola drinks, because substances such as caffeine are present in all of these, and if you continue drinking any of them you may not get a clear result. This sort of exclusion diet is simple to do, and can be very productive. At the end of about 6 days, the individual drinks should be reintroduced, but only one at a time, allowing 4 days between the tests, as they contain similar ingredients. Test them as described before, first thing in the morning on an empty stomach, taking the volume of a normal drink.

The Stone Age Diet

If you want to go on a more complicated diet, the 'Stone Age Diet', introduced by Dr R. Mackarness (author of *Not All in the Mind*) is a good one to use. This is the strictest diet we would normally recommend anyone to carry out without professional help. The Stone Age Diet can be used for two purposes: to exclude all common foods, and to exclude additives present in the diet. However, it does not exclude all the substances which get into basic foods during production, like pesticides, herbicides, and so on, although these may be reduced if organic foods are used where available. The principle is to exclude all those foods which have been introduced into the everyday diet since the end of the Stone

Age period in Man's history. Man settled at this time and started farming, and as a result he began to eat large amounts of grain and diary produce. More recently many other foodstuffs have been introduced into the diet, particularly refined foods (sugar, coffee, tea, alcohol) and a large number of additives. All these foods are left out of the Stone Age Diet, which also excludes all grains (wheat, corn, barley, oats, rye, rice, and millet) all dairy products (*see* Fig 9), tea, coffee, alcohol, all sugars and all soft drinks. In addition, chicken, eggs and citrus fruits (orange, lemon, lime, grapefruit, tangerine, and others) are left out because they are usually introduced into babies' diets too early. We also prefer to leave out nuts, as these commonly cause allergic problems.

At this point you will probably say 'What does it leave for me to eat?' In fact, it leaves a very good diet which is nutritious, except that it may be a little low in calcium. It allows all fresh meat (except chicken), including hare, rabbit, pheasant, and so on, all fresh fish, including shrimps and shellfish, all vegetables, and all fruit except citrus fruit. All these foods should be eaten fresh. Frozen foods can be eaten in moderation, provided that the packets are checked first to make sure they contain no additives, but ideally the diet should consist of fresh foods only. Any dried fruit included should be free of mineral oil or sulphur dioxide. You should avoid eating any one food to excess during the diet, especially the fruits.

You should use spring water for drinking and for cooking while you are on the diet, as foods cooked in tap water can pick up contaminating chemicals from water. Tap water contains many different chemicals (*see* Chapter 3); spring water is much better, although it may not be actually free from chemicals. Spring water should also be used for cleaning teeth.

The diet is normally followed strictly for 10 days and by the end of this time the vast majority of people who go through a with-drawal reaction are symptom-free. If you are not yet symptom-free, wait another day or two before you start testing foods. Start testing with tap water, and then go on to all the different foods that you have been avoiding during the 10-day period.

There is one other principle which is important and should be understood at this stage: that similar foods should not be tested on consecutive days. Similar foods are those that belong to the same family; a food family is made up of plants, animals, or fish that are very similar to each other, and you will find details of food families in the book by Drs Randolph and Moss. One example is the grass family which consists of wheat, corn, barley, oats, rice, rye, millet, and cane sugar. These are all basically grasses, and if you are going to test several of these you should leave 4 days between the tests. This is easy to do if you have other foods to test in the interim, as you have on the Stone Age Diet. If you test wheat on Day 2, you can test corn on Day 6, cane sugar on Day 10, oats or rice on Day 14, and barley or rye on Day 18. In between you can test the other foods you have been avoiding, being careful not to test similar foods on consective days.

Instructions for the Stone Age Diet will be found in Appendix IV: it can be used for all age groups from 2 years old to 90. In young children it is probably best to add a simple vitamin supplement (ABIDEC drops, which can be bought or prescribed, are quite sufficient) and calcium as colour-free calcium syrup, 2 teaspoons per day. Medical supervision is necessary in two groups; in babies to ensure adequate nutrition, and in young boys with eczema because of a very slight risk of anaphylaxis. We have not encountered it and only a handful of cases have been reported worldwide (none fatal) but appropriate precautions should be taken.

Other Diets

Another sort of diet you can do is one which takes out food families rather than individual foods, re-introducing them after 10 days or so (for example, a grain-free diet, or a dairy-free diet). If you do this remember to be meticulous about hidden ingredients (*see* Fig 9),and about spacing the re-introductions. In the past I (DJM) have used these, but we now usually use the Stone Age Diet because it is by far the most satisfactory diet for removing the majority of the foods that frequently cause problems, without being dangerously strict.

If you want to go on a stricter diet, or if you have been recommended to do so, it is very important that you ask either a doctor or a competent dietician to supervise what you are doing. There are various reasons for this. Firstly, you may have such a severe withdrawal reaction that you feel it necessary to call your doctor; secondly, when you start re-introducing foods you may find yourself reacting to most of them and get in a complete mess. This may result in you eating such a narrow diet that there is a significant danger of malnutrition. This applies only to the more severely affected but you can never tell at the start how bad you will prove to be. Many people would get away with a complete fast, and many health books do recommend a complete fast for one or two days. A fit person can do this and feel perfectly well, but if you suffer from significant food allergy you may become extremely ill, and barely able to cope. This is why you should always seek guidance.

Another form of diet that is commonly recommended is a rotation diet, which can be used for diagnosis or for treatment. No one should go on a 4-day rotation diet except under trained supervision because of the risk that all the essential elements of the diet will not be present in adequate quantities. For this reason it will only be mentioned here. It is a useful diet for patients who are sensitive to many foods because it helps to maintain tolerance to the foods to which they are not sensitive. It is frequently used in the long-term management of patients who are severely affected. The 4-day rotation diet makes sure that any one food is not eaten more frequently than one day in four, often only once on that day. The diet consists of numerous different foods, rigorously planned to ensure adequate nutrition, while separating foods of any one family - a job for the expert. A very good diet can be built up in this way, but it is very strict and means that your favourite cup of coffee, or tea, can only be consumed once in four days.

Although you should get specific advice from a doctor or dietician before considering a 4-day rotation diet, it is a good general principle to avoid eating the same food on consecutive days, and to widen your diet, bringing in foods you would not normally eat. This is safe, relatively easy to do, and gives some protection against the development of further food allergies, because it rules out repetitive eating.

9
Medical Treatment

DRUG TREATMENT

Traditional management of allergy problems is with drugs, and patients often have to take them for prolonged periods of time to make their symptoms tolerable. Modern drugs are invaluable in the treatment of allergic reactions, but reliance on this alone often requires the extended use of potent drugs which may result in side effects. If the responsible allergens can be identified and largely avoided, some patients may no longer need drug treatment; others (particularly the severe asthmatics) may, but the dosage required is usually much less.

Antihistamines

The baseline of medical treatment are the drugs called antihistamines. These are substances which relieve the effects of an allergic reaction by blocking the action of histamine. There are various types which differ to a certain extent in their action and potency. The earlier antihistamines all tended to have side effects, the main one being drowsiness, but more modern antihistamines cause less drowsiness and have similar potency. Their main use is to suppress itching which occurs in allergic reactions such as conjunctivitis, hay fever and rhinitis, eczema, and urticaria – the Type A allergic reactions. Antihistamines are simple to take, have relatively few side effects, and are not addictive, but it is often necessary to try out several different types before finding one that suits you. Even with the newer antihistamines, drowsiness can be a problem, particularly in people who are driving, or using dangerous machinery. Drowsiness from antihistamines can be potentiated by alcohol, so people taking them should be very careful. Some people find that the effect of antihistamines wears off after a period of time: as far as we know the reason for this is not understood.

Another difficulty, especially in children, is that antihistamines are often made up in syrups and the excipients (the extra substances added to make the preparation attractive to take, or well tolerated) can cause problems in their own right, particularly the colourings and flavourings. Even in tablets this can also be true. For a long time certain well-known antihistamines contained the colouring tartrazine, which is the azo-dye best known for causing allergic reactions.

Antihistamines are normally taken as tablets or liquids. They can also be applied on the skin but this has the disadvantage that there is a significant risk of topical sensitisation, so that the drug itself then produces an allergic reaction in the skin, making the problem worse rather than better. Antihistamines will probably always remain in the forefront of drug therapy for allergy, in view of their safety.

Intal

In the late 1960s a new substance called Di-sodium cromoglycate was discovered, and was found to have marked anti-allergic properties, again mainly in IgE-mediated reactions. It was first used in asthma as Intal, since when its use has spread to the treatment of conjunctivitis, hay fever and rhinitis. It has also been used in the treatment of food allergy, but this appears to have limited success, partly because it is often used in too small a dosage. The standard dosage recommended for food allergy is 200mg four times a day before meals; it has been found that doses up to 2g are occasionally necessary to produce a good response, and so its more widespread use has been limited by cost.

Our impression is that Intal works better in patients with Type A allergy, but we usually suggest that other patients with significant allergy problems try the drug. Sodium cromoglycate is best taken by emptying the capsules into a quarter of a cup of warm water and swilling it round the mouth for 10 seconds before swallowing it. To test its effectiveness in your case, take a high dose half an hour before eating a meal that you know will upset you and see what happens. If the drug blocks the allergic reaction, then reduce the dose successively until you find the minimum you require to produce the effect. You can then use that dose, either regularly (if you have severe allergic reactions), or before you eat out, as this is the one time that it is difficult to avoid certain foods. This drug is only available on prescription.

Intal in its various other forms is applied topically to the site of the allergic reaction – as eye-drops in allergic conjunctivitis, as a powdered or liquid aerosol intra-nasally in allergic rhinitis, and with a spinhaler or pressurised aerosol in asthma. This drug can be very effective indeed in certain patients, and is usually tried before steroids, as it has very few side effects and very rarely produces a reaction severe enough to have to stop the drug.

Steroids

Steroids are by far the most potent and effective anti-allergic preparations. They have now been available since the late 1950s and are used widely in the treatment of moderate to severe allergic reactions. Their main effect appears to be the suppression of the inflammatory response that is triggered by the reaction. They are effective in a wide range of allergic conditions, and have a profound effect on symptoms, starting within 4 to 8 hours. Patients with severe asthma or eczema, when started on a high dose, find that their symptoms rapidly disappear and they can become totally symptom-free within a few days. More severe cases do not necessarily clear completely, however high the dose.

If steroids were without side effects they would be the favoured drug for treating allergic reactions. However, like all other potent drugs they have serious side effects. These may take years to appear but when they do they may be largely irreversible. The most common reaction is thinning of the skin associated with bruising, and facial swelling and redness; the appetite is often stimulated and obesity is a common problem. Raised blood pressure, osteoporosis, recurrent infections, and diabetes can occur after long-term treatment. Diabetes only occurs in patients who are already at risk of developing the disease, but patients who are mild diabetics become much worse, and those already on insulin can have problems controlling their blood sugar if they take steroids. In children steroids may suppress growth.

Steroid preparations come in various forms, but are mostly used as tablets, since oral treatment can be effective in any form of allergic reaction. However, to try to reduce the dosage needed, and therefore the side effects, many topical preparations have been produced, such as eye drops, nasal sprays for hay fever and rhinitis, various forms of inhalers for asthma (using either powder or pressurised aerosol), and the very widely-used creams and ointments for skin conditions. Prolonged use of any of these substances may produce side effects: the safest are the preparations for the treatment of hay fever and asthma, where side effects are minimal. Preparations used in the eye can produce problems with infection and cataract formation, and those used on the skin, if used in too strong a potency, can cause wasting and thinning of the skin in the area involved. If the drug is used in large amounts it can be absorbed through the skin and produce the same side effects as oral preparations.

BIOLOGICAL TREATMENT

Desensitisation

Since the beginning of the twentieth century, attempts have been made to modify the body's reaction to allergens, as it is this which produces the symptoms. Numerous trials have been carried out, trying to make the patient 'tolerant' to the substances concerned – the terms used for this type of treatment are 'desensitisation', or 'hyposensitisation'. Desensitisation aims to stimulate the production of protective antibodies that block the allergic reaction, and involves the injection of increasing doses of the allergen. Until quite recently, desensitisation to grass pollen and house dust mite was used quite widely, and desensitisation was also used in certain cases of animal allergies and in the treatment of bee and wasp sting allergy.

Although controlled trials had shown that desensitisation was definitely effective in hay fever, house dust mite allergy, and some cases of animal allergy, there were a number of problems associated with this sort of treatment. Side effects were not uncommon, and occasionally fatal reactions would occur, especially in patients who were suffering from asthma. There was no formal education for the doctors or paramedical staff carrying out desensitisation, and so treatment was somewhat haphazard. There were also problems with the preparation and standardisation of the antigens used, and with correct identification of the specific antigen causing the patient's symptoms. Too much reliance was placed on skin test results rather than on history or blood tests. As a result, many patients were desensitised to substances that were not actually causing problems and too many substances were included in each course of desensitisation, reducing the effectiveness. In the 1980s these problems started to be solved, with the development of techniques for purifying the antigens and improved diagnosis in the individual patient.

In 1986 the Committee for Safety of Medicines (CSM), following an investigation into the deaths of patients who were being treated by desensitisation, made very strict recommendations about the minimum conditions under which desensitisation could be carried out. As a result of their report, desensitisation has virtually been withdrawn as a treatment in this country. Its use is now limited to relatively few centres, and is almost entirely hospital-based: the UK is now the only country in the Western world where desensitisation is hardly ever used. A knock-on effect which is causing concern is that the allergy preparations used are now difficult to obtain in the UK for testing, as desensitisation provided their main market.

Neutralisation

Other treatments have also been developed to try and modify the patient's reaction to the allergen. One of these, developed in the USA, is termed 'neutralisation'. In the early 1960s Dr Carlton Lee and Dr Rinkel, working with desensitisation, found that a very low dose of the antigen produced just as good an effect as a high dose. As a result of this discovery the technique of neutralisation has gradually been developed and is now used by a significant number of doctors in the USA and a few in the UK.

The technique involves testing the patient to find the dilution of the antigen which just fails to cause any reaction, either in the skin or in the body generally. Injection of a very small volume of this dilution, or absorption of the same dilution from under the tongue, produces relief from allergic symptoms caused by that allergen (and that allergen alone) for a period varying from a few hours to two or more days. Once the dose is established it is kept constant, and, because it is individually titrated for each patient, it is not normally associated with any side effects. The patients are taught to give their own injections (usually every other day), or their sub-lingual drops (taken more frequently). The mode of action of neutralisation is not understood, but it was shown to be effective in a double-blind trial at the Middlesex Hospital, London. We have many patients who are able to take a much wider diet, and/or be exposed to inhalants or chemicals without symptoms while on neutralisation, but get symptoms without it. On this sort of regime many patients keep more or less symptom-free without drug treatment.

Enzyme-Potentiated Desensitisation

Another technique, which has been developed in the UK, by Dr Len McEwan working at St Mary's Hospital, Paddington, London, is Enzyme-Potentiated Desensitisation or EPD. This again is only available in a few centres in the UK at the moment. The technique is relatively simple, and consists of mixing the appropriate antigens with a naturally-occurring enzyme, beta-glucuronidase, and either injecting them or placing them in a small plastic cup which is applied to the forearm for 24 hours over an area from which the superficial layers of the skin have been removed. The treatment has been found capable of re-establishing tolerance in 1–2 years, giving treatment at intervals of from 1–3 months; for best results there should also be appropriate control of diet. Research studies have shown that it is effective in hay fever, eczema and other conditions, and it is hoped that in due course the technique will become more widely available, and better recognised.

Nystatin

In recent years there have been reports suggesting that gross infection of the gut with *Candida albicans* (the organism that causes thrush) can cause symptoms very similar to those caused by allergies. A number of doctors seem to get very good results from an anti-*Candida* regime involving the use of nystatin (in pure powder form) or another drug, and a diet restricting carbohydrates, yeast-containing foods, fungi and sometimes fruit – a diet which also removes some of the most troublesome allergens. In our experience, most patients respond well to intensive allergy management and few seem to need anti-*Candida* treatment in addition.

Homoeopathy

For a long time homoeopathic remedies have been used in the treatment of allergic conditions. In 1987 the first controlled trial of homoeopathic treatment in hay fever was published from Glasgow; it showed that homoeopathy was significantly more effective than placebo in treating this condition. The paper was received with considerable scepticism by the medical profession, but further trials are in hand to confirm the efficacy of homoeopathy in allergic conditions, and it may, in the future, become another recognised treatment.

Nutritional Medicine

Nutrition is a major factor in the management of allergic conditions. For many years practitioners using the nutritional approach have claimed good results in patients suffering from allergies. The evidence suggests that this is quite logical. Relatively recently various studies have shown that the assumption that the modern diet has adequate amounts of the various essential nutrients, including the various vitamins and minerals, may not be correct. Intensive farming practices favour the progressive reduction in trace mineral content in the soil, in its vegetable products, and of the stock fed on them. Delays from the harvesting of crops to arrival in the shops lead to substantial loss of vitamin content, and that loss is increased by some of the treatments used to preserve the crops during transport. Further losses occur when foods are prepared hours before consumption: this is now much more common than it used to be in restaurants, canteens, and in the home, especially with pre-packed and convenience foods. There are additional losses of both vitamins and minerals when vegetables are over-cooked, or cooked in too large a volume of water, or if the cooking water is discarded; these are all errors common in the UK.

An increasing number of studies are now being published showing that marginal deficiencies of various vitamins and minerals may be far more common than previously thought. For instance, in the UK it has been shown that up to 50 per cent of elderly patients being admitted to hospital may have evidence of vitamin C deficiency, and sub-clinical deficiencies of other vitamins as well. At present too little is known about nutrition to be certain exactly what effect these deficiencies would have in the development of allergic problems. It is known that several of these substances are essential for immune reactions; some are used up during the reaction, others seem to be needed if the immune system is to function properly. It therefore seems logical to assume that patients who are mildly deficient in certain vitamins and minerals have reduced ability to recover from illness, or from allergic reactions, and that impaired control of immune reactions due to mild deficiency might contribute to the development of allergic disease. Correcting this by giving the appropriate nutritional supplements could then be expected to contribute to recovery.

The human body is remarkably resilient and given the correct conditions can recover from even very serious illness. There is no reason to assume that patients cannot recover from allergic problems; indeed, it is our experience that some patients do recover with good management. The use of appropriate nutritional supplements seems to play a part in this improvement: some patients improve on supplementation, and relapse when it is stopped. You will find a fuller treatment of this subject in *Nutritional Medicine* by Drs Davies and Stewart (Pan Books, 1987).

It seems that minor deficiencies of both vitamins and minerals are exacerbated by allergic reactions, and that they in turn delay recovery. We are sufficiently convinced of this to recommend supplementation with both to many of our patients, but there is a need for further research.

10
Your Health in Your Hands

Having read as far as this, you will have become aware that there are a multitude of different substances which can cause adverse reactions through allergy, intolerance, or pseudo-allergy, but that the amount of distress that is caused by them varies widely. At one extreme there are many people who are upset by just one or two substances, who recognise the fact, avoid these substances and have no more problems. However, at the other end there are people who react to many different things and have intractable symptoms; they may even be so disabled that it is impossible for them to lead a normal life. Why does this happen? A good way to look at this is in terms of blocks piling up to a give a total load. This is illustrated in Fig 10. The individual building blocks refer to specific allergens to which the patient is responding; they are grouped together as inhalants, chemicals and foods. The threshold is the level at which the allergic individual develops symptoms.

The first column shows someone who is exposed to a moderate amount of a large number of allergens, and the total load exceeds the threshold by a small amount: you will notice that if any of the building blocks are removed the total load drops below the threshold and the patient becomes symptom-free. For these patients minor variations in environmental exposure can make the difference between being symptom-free and symptomatic. For instance, the patient who is sensitive to grass pollen may only have symptoms during the summer. This may be the case not only for symptoms directly related to pollen exposure, but also symptoms from foods; they may not be able to eat certain foods during the summer although they can eat them during the winter. Another example is a patient who owns a pet; if it dies he may become symptom-free within two or three months, as the allergen level drops. It may appear that all their troubles were due to the pet, whereas the important factor may have been the contribution the pet made to the total allergen level. This has quite different implications for necessary future precautions.

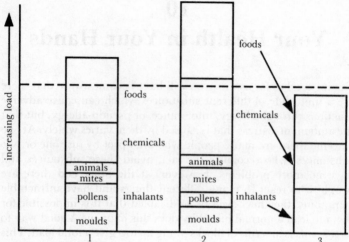

Fig 10   Total allergen load and the development of symptoms.

The second column shows someone exposed to a much higher level of allergens. Here, removal of only one building block will make no difference to their symptoms, so all three groups of allergens may need to be substantially reduced to make any real improvement, as shown in the third column.

The threshold at which any patient will produce symptoms is not fixed and various factors influence it. This is shown in Fig 11 The threshold can be raised by all the factors that promote good health; specifically by good stress management (using any of the techniques that promote relaxation), making sure that your nutrition is more than adequate, and having a full and satisfying life. The threshold is lowered by many factors, but the main ones are stress, infection and poor nutrition. If you go back to Fig 10, you will see the influence of the threshold on the development of symptoms. The more you can raise your threshold, the less likely you are to develop symptoms, or the more easily symptoms will be controlled if you already have them. Any drop in threshold may produce an acute exacerbation of your symptoms. When this happens, it is not necessarily due to an increase in exposure, but could just as easily be due to a change in threshold.

Let us run through the various influences. Firstly, there is the

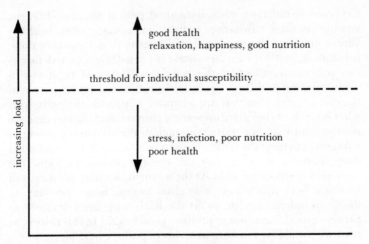

Fig 11   Factors affecting the threshold of symptoms.

degree of sensitivity to the allergen: the cause of this sensitivity is not fully understood, except that we know genetic predisposition plays an important part, and that an initial exposure to the allergen is essential; the *size* of that initial exposure may be critical. We also know that certain precipitating factors – infections (particularly viral infections), toxic chemical exposure, operations, and severe unavoidable stress – may lead to sensitisation to whatever allergens were about at the time. For instance, gastro-enteritis increases the likelihood of developing allergy to foods eaten at that time. In each case the patient may suddenly become allergic. So these factors have two effects: they *increase* the likelihood of the patient becoming allergic, and for the allergic patient they *increase* the likelihood of developing symptoms, by lowering the threshold. Certain hormonal effects, including puberty, meno-pause, pregnancy and the contraceptive pill, also tend to alter the threshold at which an individual patient gets symptoms, usually lowering it, although pregnancy may affect it either way.

Of the other general factors that can affect the threshold, probably the most under-recognised is nutrition. The body re-quires four major groups of substances to function normally – vitamins, minerals, essential fatty acids and essential aminoacids.

Everyone is different; each individual person requires different amounts of these substances to function normally when healthy. Illness increases the requirements for some (if not most) of these substances, and if the dietary intake is not sufficient then deficiencies will occur, affecting the body's capability of coping with environmental problems. Essential nutrients may not be present in the diet in quantities that are adequate to provide the body with what it needs. Articles are appearing emphasising the fact that the modern diet may not contain enough of the recognised essential substances to meet the basic requirements (termed 'recommended daily intakes', or 'RDIs') of the average person, let alone the increased needs of the sick. At the moment, we have no means of knowing how much any individual person needs per day to maintain optimal health; so far the RDIs have been designed to prevent gross illness, not to produce good health. In this respect at least we should be thinking in terms of positive health.

For good nutrition, attention used to be focused mainly on ensuring an adequate intake of protein and of some of the vitamins, but the importance of many of the minerals has become increasingly apparent, and recently attention has focused on the essential fatty acids. These fall into two groups – the omega-3 fatty acids (the ones present in fish oils) which have recently been in the news as protective factors in relation to coronary heart disease, and the omega-6 fatty acids (in evening primrose oil and some other vegetable oils) which improve menstrual disorders and eczema, and may well be helpful in other allergic diseases. The importance of many of the substances that are now recognised as being essential was not apparent in the 1960s and there may be other factors yet to be discovered. In *Nutritional Medicine* Drs Davies and Stewart (*see* Further Reading) give a full discussion of the present position, but if you think you are deficient you should seek professional help.

The other main factor is general health. If the patient has any other illness or is being treated with drugs this inevitably affects the functioning of the rest of the body adversely, reducing the threshold. Emotional stress can also play a major part, as one of the major effects of stress is on the immune system; this reduces the body's capability of coping with other environmental stresses. Experiments in animals and experience with man show that it is unavoidable stress that has the most marked effect; the sort of stress that makes you feel powerless and hopeless. If you are under stress, make an effort to learn about good stress management. Use some sort of relaxation or meditation technique regularly and take regular exercise. These will all tend to counter the effects of a stressful life. Finally, it would probably be worth spending a little time thinking about your life, about the things that you find deeply satisfying, and about how to organise your time to make sure that these things are not squeezed out. Being happy and fulfilled will raise the threshold, just as being self-absorbed and miserable tends to lower it.

Why does it matter if you have symptoms? Partly, of course, because it is unpleasant and may be disabling. But the main reason is that while you are reacting to allergens you will be more likely to develop further allergies. Occasional reactions are not important, but reacting continuously or very frequently is likely to make you progressively worse. In contrast, if you are well your body has a chance of recuperating and overcoming the allergies with a return of tolerance to modest exposures.

This brings us to another concept, the difference between allergy and allergic disease, best illustrated using the bath as a model (Fig 12). This time the allergen load is represented by the pressure in each of the three taps – inhalants, foods, and chemicals. In allergic people the taps are turned on, and the amount they are turned on is determined by the degree of sensitivity. The outlet is the person's ability to cope, and it makes a major contribution to determining the threshold. If the pressure is very low the water will all be able to

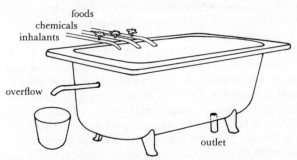

Fig 12   Symptoms as the overflow of water building up in a bath.

run away, even if the taps are full on. If the rate of the water flowing in exceeds the capacity of the outlet, the bath will slowly fill up. The body has considerable reserves and for some time nothing will happen. When the bath fills to the top and overflows the patient develops symptoms; the greater the overflow, the worse the symptoms. Normally both the patient and the doctors assume that the illness has started at this time, when in fact things may have been going wrong for months or years beforehand; it is only when the bath overflows that the symptoms occur. Looking back you may realise that there have been periods in the past when it had happened before, when there were similar symptoms for short periods which apparently cleared spontaneously with or without treatment. This may date back as far as childhood in some people.

Commonly people are unwell when they are very young and grow out of it between the ages of 5 and 20 years of age. They may then seem well for a variable period of time (anything from a few months to 50 or 60 years) before their symptoms recur. It seems likely that in these patients the overflow simply stopped for this period (presumably because as they grew they developed more ability to cope), and then came back again as they got older. Asthmatics classically show this pattern; a child who suffers from asthma appears to grow out of the asthma by about 10 or 12 years of age and then is symptom-free until 40 or 50, when the asthma returns for the rest of his life. With careful questioning, such sufferers often admit that they had very mild attacks of asthma in between (usually precipitated by exercise or illnesses), which were not bad enough for them to go to the doctor, and never bad enough to worry about. These illnesses represent periods when the bath was overflowing under extra stress, but not enough to cause significant problems.

The period when the patient is symptom-free but hatching trouble is potentially very important. Anyone who was aware of the situation might well take care to avoid repeated excess exposure, and do everything in their power to increase their threshold to stave off the onset of symptoms. However, if they think they are well, there is no reason to take any preventive action.

When the overflow starts the patient develops symptoms, and this is the onset of the illness as far as the medical profession is concerned. Modern medicine basically treats the overflow with medication, which is represented in the illustration by the bucket placed under the overflow. The more potent the medication, the larger the bucket; the more often it is taken, the more frequently the bucket is replaced. You can see that a potent medication taken often will be highly effective at keeping the floor dry, while a less potent medication taken less frequently will be far less effective, simply reducing the size of the puddle (the severity of the symptoms), but not containing all the overflow. If you look at the diagram as a whole, you will realise that the drug treatment approach ignores the cause of the symptoms; it is merely an exercise in damage-limitation.

Managing allergies entails tackling all aspects in order to deal with *all* the allergens to which you are reacting. For some people it may mean doing something about diet, about features in the home that encourage mites or moulds, about personal habits and about the use of chemicals. Others may only have to make minor modifications to one of these areas (though they would be wise to cut down the use of chemicals as well, as a precaution). The results are often extremely rewarding: people are continually telling us that since they made the changes they have felt well and active for the first time in years. Most people find that the restrictions needed are well worth while, and keep to them strictly most of the time, realising (often for the first time) that bodies should be comfortable, and that symptoms are the body's way of demanding that we change our ways.

This book has been mainly concerned with helping you to look at your environment, and to identify as many causes as possible which you yourself can either avoid or modify. It has pointed to things you can do yourself to increase your body's ability to cope, but for specific treatment you have to rely on professional help. As knowledge of allergy and of nutrition grows, it is to be hoped that better management in these respects will become much more widely available. Drug treatment is important and has produced dramatic improvements in the management of many illnesses, but we must stop relying on more and more potent drugs and find the basic cause of the problems. For instance, in recurrent infections of any sort (common in allergics, particularly in children) antibiotics are used very widely and very frequently. In the USA one figure quoted is that all children under about 5 years of age have a course of antibiotics every 4 to 6 weeks: under these circumstances the doctor is exposing the child to repeated courses of potent drugs with the inevitable risk of side effects, instead of looking to see why the child is having infections. It is vitally important that a cause should be looked for in patients who suffer in this way. The two commonest (and most freqently overlooked) reasons for this happening are probably poor nutrition and allergy.

Hopefully as time goes on the medical profession will become much more aware of the effect that the environment and nutrition can have on the individual person, and take a more holistic approach to the treatment of medical conditions. This already appears to be happening and there are signs that it may be gathering momentum, but it is impossible to say how long it will be before the majority of doctors take this view. In the meantime as there are so few doctors who are interested in this field, patients will have to create the conditions under which change will occur. You can put pressure on your doctors, influencing them to take notice of these new trends, you can combine with others to make sure that those responsible for health services know of deficiencies, and you can put your own house in order, taking responsibility for your own health, especially in relation to smoking, alcohol consumption, drugs, poor eating habits, and exposure to chemicals. All of these can affect your health adversely and in the long term cause major problems, even serious illness. Lastly, you can take all possible precautions to protect the next generation, and influence others to do the same, in an attempt to stop the increasing epidemic of allergic disease.

Appendices

I ADDRESSES OF ORGANISATIONS
(Please send a stamped addressed envelope (SAE) with enquiries.)

Airedale Allergy Centre
High Hall
Steeton
Nr Keighley
West Yorkshire BD20 6SB

Action Against Allergy
43 The Downs
London SW20 8HG

Allergy Patients Support Groups
(Register)
c/o PO Box 24
Skipton
North Yorkshire BD23 6QG

Asthma Society and Friends of
    Asthma Research Council
St Thomas's Hospital
Lambeth Palace Road
London SE1 7EH

British Association of Nurses
    in Allergy and Environmental
    Medicine
P.O. Box 24
Skipton
North Yorkshire BD23 6QG

British Society for Allergy and
    Environmental Medicine
'Acorns'
Romsey Road
Southampton SO4 2NN

British Society for Allergy and
    Clinical Immunology
Dept of Respiratory Medicine
St Bartholomew's Hospital
London EC1A 7BE

Coeliac Society
P.O. Box 220
High Wycombe
Buckinghamshire HP11 2HY

Foresight: The Association for
    the Promotion of
    Preconceptual Care
Mrs Barnes
The Old Vicarage
Church Lane, Witley
Godalming
Surrey GU8 5PN

The Henry Doubleday Research Association (organic growing methods)
Ryton-on-Dunsmore
Coventry
Warwickshire CV8 3LG

Hyperactive Childen's Support Group
71 Wyke Lane
Chichester
West Sussex PO19 2LD

McCarrison Society (nutrition and health)
24 Paddington Street
London W1M 4DR

Myalgic Encephalomyelitis (M.E.) Association
P.O. Box 8
Stanford-Le-Hope
Essex IG3 8NF

National Eczema Society
Tavistock House East
Tavistock Square
London WC1H 9SR

National Society for Research in Allergy
P.O. Box 45
Hinckley
Leicestershire LE10 1JY

II SUPPLIERS

The vacuum cleaner mentioned in the text (Medivac) can be obtained from Taylormaid Products Ltd (Tel: 0625 827922). Hypoallergenic products marketed by Amway UK Ltd (Tel: 0908 679888) and Shaklee UK Ltd (0908 660655) are available through agents: Ecover, Boots, Almay, and Simple products are available through retail outlets including health food shops and chemists. Health food shops carry a range of untreated dried fruits and other foods: foods (and some equipment) can be purchased mail order from Food-Watch International, Butts Pond Industrial Estate, Sturminster Newton, Dorset DT10 1AZ (send SAE for list). Wide-ranging and up-dated lists of products and suppliers can be obtained from the Airedale Allergy Centre (foods, clothing, bedding, and all other products referred to in the text), the National Eczema Society (personal toiletries, clothing, etc), and Action Against Allergy; for addresses *see* Appendix I. In each case please enclose three first-class stamps to cover costs.

III Food Challenge Chart

Name . . . .

Challenge Sheet No . . . .

DATE	WEIGHT		RESTING PULSE RATE	TIME	FOOD TESTED	RESTING PULSE AFTER			NOTES ON REACTIONS OCCURRING AND TIME
	AM	PM				20 mins	40 mins	60 mins	

IV STONE AGE DIET
(After Dr R. Mackarness)

The Guidelines

1. Before you start your diet, reduce your exposure to chemicals to a minimum. Replace essential toiletries with simple and non-perfumed products. Avoid the use of air-fresheners or aerosols: keep to simple chemical cleaning compounds.
2. Avoid toothpaste – use sodium bicarbonate or a 2:1 mixture of sea salt and sodium bicarbonate instead.
3. Avoid all drugs bought over the counter, cigarettes and all other tobacco products, and alcohol. Drugs, drinks and tobacco products are frequently the cause of allergic reactions. You *must* avoid them.
4. Avoid taking prescribed drugs unless this is inadvisable on medical grounds: if in doubt discuss it with your doctor.
5. Avoid all processed and packaged foods: these contain preservatives, flavourings, colourings, additives etc., and are refined and processed to the detriment of their nutritional content. Start to read the contents of packaged foods. Be sure to avoid:

> All tinned and packaged foods
> Processed and convenience foods (crisps, snacks, etc)
> Lemonade, fruit squashes, fizzy drinks, etc
> Margarine, sweets, chocolates, all cereals
> Processed meats, gravy, sauces

6. Avoid the main foods that cause allergies:

> Milk, cream, cheese, butter, yoghurt and other dairy products
> Wheat, corn, all other grains and cereals
> Chicken, eggs
> Tea, coffee, chocolate, sugar
> Citrus fruit

Remember – no bread, no biscuits, no cakes, etc

What You Can Eat

You can eat *any fresh meat*, except for chicken; *any fresh fish*; *any fresh fruit*, except for citrus fruits (such as orange, lemon, lime, grapefruit); *any fresh vegetables* (including potatoes, root vegetables, leafy greens, etc); *dried fruit* (untreated); *sea salt*. Try varieties you do not normally have. Experiment with these fresh foods in different combinations and widen your eating habits. Choose organic foods when available. If fresh food is in short supply use good quality frozen vegetables without additives.

Any cooking method – boiling, frying, stewing, grilling, roasting – can be used, but use sunflower, safflower or olive oil (preferably cold-pressed) or meat fat, and use bottled spring water. Do not use corn or vegetable oils. This means you can have chips and any other fresh food fried if you wish; there is no need to be hungry as there is no limit to the *quantity* that can be eaten.

What You Can Drink

Bottled spring water is best. For extra variety try herb teas, preferably not tea-bags; the paper is processed in formaldehyde. Try to use several different kinds.

Fruit juices (unsweetened with no preservative) are safe *in moderation*. Use grape, apple and pineapple (not citrus juices) – dilute them at least half and half, as they are very concentrated. Try vegetable juices (bottled or home-made).

Persevere

Keep to this regime as strictly as you can for 10 days. Remember that if you feel worse at first you really *needed* to do the diet. When the going seems tough (as it often does) remember that the best way to sort out your allergy is to have this period without exposure to any of the common food allergens. Keeping to this strictly gives you the best chance of a good result. After 5–6 days you will probably be starting to feel better and by 10 days be ready to start re-introducing foods.

If your symptoms do not change during the Stone Age Diet, it is unlikely that food allergy is your problem and you should go back on to a normal diet.

If you get worse initially on the diet but are not improving after 7 days, count the number of times you have been eating each individual food while on the diet; stay on the diet for a further week but leave out the two foods you have been eating most frequently, and avoid water from plastic bottles and plastic-wrapped food. If you do not then improve, go back on to a normal diet: you should not try any further dietary restrictions without expert guidance.

Re-Introduction

After completing the initial 10 days on the Stone Age Diet, you should test the foods you have been avoiding. Make yourself a chart (*see* Appendix III) on which to record your reactions and do *one test* each day. First test your home water, then proceed to test foods in the following order: milk (½ pint), wholemeal bread, tea, cheese (white), eggs (2), sweetcorn, coffee (ground), butter, chicken, cane sugar (Tate & Lyle), chocolate (plain), citrus fruit, beet sugar (Silver Spoon), oats or rice, food colourings (1 tsp each of 4), monosodium glutamate (E621–3, packet soups), margarine, barley or rye, alcohol. Take the food at breakfast-time and make sure you have a large helping of it. The food should be taken again at lunch-time and tea-time if no reactions have occurred.

Weigh yourself morning and evening on each test day and take your resting pulse rate before testing the food and 20, 40 and 60 minutes afterwards. If you get symptoms, you have reacted, but a pulse rise or fall of more than 10 beats per minute or a weight gain of more than 1 lb (½kg) over the day also indicates a reaction.

You should remain on the basic diet until you have tested all the foods on the list: once you have tested them all you can re-introduce the foods to which you did not react, leaving out the foods that caused reactions of any kind. You should then proceed to test any additional foods which you wish to eat, and to re-test any foods which gave inconclusive results.

The Stone Age Diet is nutritious and adequate for most people even over a longer period, but if you react to many foods it is wise to discuss your remaining diet with your doctor or dietician.

V GLOSSARY

Antigen/allergen A substance that induces and elicits an immune response. The two terms are often used interchangeably though the response to an allergen is usually harmful to the body.

Atopic A term used for individuals who have a tendency to overproduce IgE and develop allergic disease.

Challenge The process of exposing a person to an allergen (food, inhalant or chemical, etc.) or a substance to which they may be intolerant, and observing the reaction. The challenge may be by mouth, by inhalation or by touch.

Intolerance Strictly a biochemcial idiosyncracy, an inbuilt anomaly (usually of an enzyme) which results in the failure of, or abnormal products from, the breakdown of certain substances in the body: either the original substance, or one of the products may then be toxic. The term is often used for any other abnormal response.

Less allergenic/more allergenic Concerned with the ease with which a substance invokes an allergic reaction, mainly dependent on chemical structure and configuration.

Mediators Chemical substances that transmit messages within the body; they are involved in bringing about the effects of allergic reactions and nerve activity, etc.

Neutralisation The use of individually-titrated, very low doses of an allergen to block the allergic reaction of the body to that allergen.

Pseudo-allergic That which mimics an allergic reaction, but is triggered by a chemical, not an allergic, reaction.

Specificity The 'fit' between antigen (allergen) and antibody which is the basic characteristic of the immune response. Antigen and antibody will only react when they have the same specificity.

Syndrome A collection of symptoms occurring together.

Topical Applied locally, to skin, eyes, etc.

Volatile The essence of a solid or liquid substance that enters the air in the gaseous phase; for instance the ability to smell perfume, or the scent of a rose, depends on volatilisation of the essence of each.

VI FURTHER READING

Davies, S. and Stewart, A. *Nutritional Medicine* (Pan Books, 1987)

Faelten, S. *The Allergy Self-Help Book* (Rodale Press, 1983)

Golos, N. and Golos Goldblitz, F. *Coping with your Allergies* (Simon & Schuster, 1986)

Hannsen, M. *New E for Additives* (Thorsons, 1987)

Kingsley, P. *Conquering Cystitis* (Ebury Press, 1987)

Levin, A.S. and Zellerbach, M. *The Allergy Relief Programme* (Gateway Books, 1983)

London Food Commission, *Food Adulteration and How to Beat It* (Unwin, 1988)

Mackarness, R. *Not All in the Mind* (Pan Books, 1976)

Mansfield, J. *The Migraine Revolution* (Thorsons, 1986)

Minchen, M. *Food for Thought, A Parent's Guide to Food Intolerance* (O.U.P., 1986)

Pottenger, F.M. Jr. *Pottenger's Cats, a Study in Nutrition* (Price-Pottenger Nutrition Foundation Inc., 1983)

Randolph, T.G. and Moss, R.W. *Allergies, Your Hidden Enemy* (Thorsons, 1981)

Rapp, D.J. *The Impossible Child* (Practical Allergy Research Association, 1986)

Rousseau, D., Rea, W.J. and Enwright, J. *Your Home, Your Health, and Well-Being* (Hartley & Marks, 1987)

Schauss, A. *Diet, Crime and Delinquency* (Parker House, Berkeley, 1981)

Zamm, A.V. *Why Your House May Endanger Your Health* (Simon & Schuster, 1980)